Implementation of Therapeutic Hypothermia in Medicine

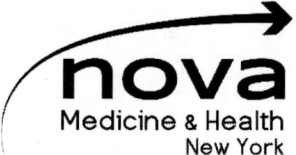

Human Anatomy and Physiology Series

Textbook of Clinical Embryology
Pranav Kumar Prabhakar, PhD, Sandeep Sharma, PhD and Manish Vyas, PhD (Editors)
eBook ISBN: 979-8-89113-317-4

The Forebrain: Development, Physiology and Functions
Morten F. Thorsen (Editor)
ISBN: 978-1-53618-407-5
eBook ISBN: 978-1-53618-426-6

The Role of Essential Metals in Human Nutrition
Andreas M. Grabrucker, PhD
ISBN: 979-8-88697-781-3
eBook ISBN: 979-8-89113-032-6

The Temporomandibular Joint: Structure, Function and Clinical Significance
Jordon Conrad (Editor)
eBook ISBN: 978-1-53617-441-0

Circadian Clock: Regulations, Genetic and External Factors
Nathaniel Hayes (Editor)
ISBN: 978-1-53613-372-1
eBook ISBN: 978-1-53613-373-8

Molecular Signaling of Mammalian Inner Ear Development
Dorothy A. Frenz (Editor)
ISBN: 978-1-62618-992-8
eBook ISBN: 978-1-62808-000-1

Anthropometry: Types, Uses and Applications
Sébastien Legrand (Editor)
ISBN: 978-1-53619-269-8
eBook ISBN: 978-1-53619-293-3

More information about this series can be found at
https://novapublishers.com/product-category/series/human-anatomy-and-physiology/

Hassan Soleimanpour
Tannaz Novinbahador
Farzad Rahmani

Implementation of Therapeutic Hypothermia in Medicine

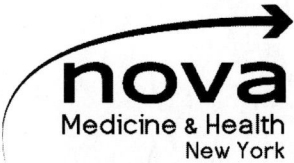

Copyright © 2025 by Nova Science Publishers, Inc.
DOI: https://doi.org/10.52305/JOGG4137

All rights reserved. No part of this book may be reproduced, stored in a retrieval system or transmitted in any form or by any means: electronic, electrostatic, magnetic, tape, mechanical photocopying, recording or otherwise without the written permission of the Publisher.

We have partnered with Copyright Clearance Center to make it easy for you to obtain permissions to reuse content from this publication. Simply navigate to this publication's page on Nova's website and locate the "Get Permission" button below the title description. This button is linked directly to the title's permission page on copyright.com. Alternatively, you can visit copyright.com and search by title, ISBN, or ISSN.

For further questions about using the service on copyright.com, please contact:
Copyright Clearance Center
Phone: +1-(978) 750-8400   Fax: +1-(978) 750-4470   E-mail: info@copyright.com.

NOTICE TO THE READER

The Publisher has taken reasonable care in the preparation of this book, but makes no expressed or implied warranty of any kind and assumes no responsibility for any errors or omissions. No liability is assumed for incidental or consequential damages in connection with or arising out of information contained in this book. The Publisher shall not be liable for any special, consequential, or exemplary damages resulting, in whole or in part, from the readers' use of, or reliance upon, this material. Any parts of this book based on government reports are so indicated and copyright is claimed for those parts to the extent applicable to compilations of such works.

Independent verification should be sought for any data, advice or recommendations contained in this book. In addition, no responsibility is assumed by the Publisher for any injury and/or damage to persons or property arising from any methods, products, instructions, ideas or otherwise contained in this publication.

The Publisher assumes no responsibility for any statements of fact or opinion expressed in the published contents.

This publication is designed to provide accurate and authoritative information with regard to the subject matter covered herein. It is sold with the clear understanding that the Publisher is not engaged in rendering legal or any other professional services. If legal or any other expert assistance is required, the services of a competent person should be sought. FROM A DECLARATION OF PARTICIPANTS JOINTLY ADOPTED BY A COMMITTEE OF THE AMERICAN BAR ASSOCIATION AND A COMMITTEE OF PUBLISHERS.

Additional color graphics may be available in the e-book version of this book.

Library of Congress Cataloging-in-Publication Data

ISBN: 979-8-89530-688-8 (Softcover)
ISBN: 979-8-89530-723-6 (eBook)

Published by Nova Science Publishers, Inc. † New York

Dedicated to:

*Professor Peter Saffer (May his soul rest in peace),
pioneer in the science of therapeutic hypothermia
for cardiac arrest patients*

*Professor Wilhelm Behringer,
former professor at the medical university of Vienna
and current professor at the university of Jena*

*Dr. Changiz Gholipouri (May his soul rest in peace),
founder of the department of emergency medicine,
Tabriz university of medical sciences, Iran*

*All the dedicated doctors, nurses, and staff in the emergency
and intensive care units who tirelessly strive and sacrifice to save
the lives of those in need*

Contents

Preface		xiii
Acknowledgments		xv
Introduction and History		xvii
Abbreviations		xix
Chapter 1	Review of the Literature	1
Chapter 2	**The Mechanism of Action of Therapeutic Hypothermia**	5
	Brain Metabolism	6
	Apoptosis, Calpain-Related Proteolysis, and Mitochondrial Dysfunction	6
	Ion Pumps and Neuronal Excitation Associated with Cardiac Arrest	6
	Immune Response	7
	Free Radicals	8
	Vascular Permeability, Blood-Brain Barrier Damage, and Edema Formation	8
	Intracellular and Extracellular Acidosis-Brain Metabolism	9
	Brain Temperature	9
	Coagulative Activity	10
	Factors Affecting the Vessels	10
	Ischemic Tolerance	11
	Seizure Activity and Other Factors	11
Chapter 3	**The Side Effects of Therapeutic Hypothermia**	13
	Arrhythmia, Hemodynamic Changes, and Cardiovascular Effects	14
	Coronary Blood Flow and Ischemia	15

viii Contents

	Electrolyte Disturbances...16
	Hyperglycemia 17
	Other Metabolic Effects and Blood Gas Levels 17
	Coagulation System..18
	Infection..18
	The Risk of Infection Associated with Therapeutic Hypothermia...19
	Preventing Infection in Hypothermic Patients................22
	Shivering...22
	Other Side Effects...23
Chapter 4	**Inclusion and Exclusion Criteria for Hypothermia Implementation**...................................25
Chapter 5	**Patient Sedation and Analgesia** 27
	Opiates..27
	Meperidine.. *27*
	Morphine *27*
	Fentanyl.. *28*
	Remifentanil... *28*
	Sufentanil... *29*
	Sedatives...29
	Midazolam... *29*
	Propofol... *30*
	Muscle Relaxants..31
	Pancuronium *31*
	Atracurium... *31*
	Vecuronium *32*
	Cisatracurium.. *32*
Chapter 6	**Initial Patient Assessment** 35
	Airway and Breathing...35
	Applications for Capnography Encompass 36
	Blood Circulation 37
	The Steps to Be Taken Before Initiating Hypothermia 37
	Core Temperature Measurement 38
	Measuring the Depth of Anesthesia: Bispectral Index (BIS)..38
Chapter 7	**Induction of Therapeutic Hypothermia**........................41
	Types of Cooling Methods 41

Surface Cooling *41*
High Volume of Intravenous Cold Fluid *42*
Intravascular Cooling *43*
Cardiopulmonary Bypass and
Extracorporeal Membrane Oxygenation *44*
Trans Nasal Cooling Device (RhinoChill) *44*
Pharmacological Techniques *44*
Ice-Cold Perfluorocarbon Ventilation *45*
Body Cavity Lavage *46*
Ventilation in aCooled
Perfluorocarbon Environment *46*
Lavage of Body Cavities *47*
Brain Cooling Alone *47*
Time to Start Cooling *47*
Rate and Duration of Cooling *48*
Maintenance of Hypothermia *48*
Targeted Temperature Management 48
Contraindications for Targeted
Temperature Management 49
Temperature Control After In-Hospital
Cardiac Arrest 50

Chapter 8   **Patient Rewarming Protocol** 53
Patient Rewarming Guide 53
Summary 53

Chapter 9   **The Implementation of Hypothermia**
in Cardiac Arrest 55
Pathophysiology of Neuronal Injury
in Cardiac Arrest 55
Pathophysiology of Neuronal Damage
in Cardiac Arrest 57
Mechanism of Hypothermia 57
Cooling of the Body Surface 58
When Should Cooling Be Initiated? 58
Potential Risks Associated with Cooling Methods 59
Large Volume of Intravenous Cold Fluids 60
Intravascular Cooling 60

Chapter 10	**Therapeutic Hypothermia in Myocardial Infraction**	61
	Critical Period for Hypothermia Management	62
	Types of Hypothermia Induction after MI	62
	Impact of Therapeutic Hypothermia on Infarct Reduction	63
	Clinical Trials	64
	Possible Mechanism of TH After MI	65
	Hypothermia Causes Energy Preservation	66
	The Effect of Hypothermia Implementation on Mitochondria and Reactive Oxygen Species	67
	The Effect of Hypothermia on Signaling Pathways	68
	The Effect of Therapeutic Hypothermia on Microvascular Obstruction	68
	TH for Cardiogenic Shock Associated with STEMI	69
	Potential Reasons for Lack of Efficacy in Clinical Trials	69
	Future Directions	70
	Conclusion	70
Chapter 11	**Hypothermia Implementation in Acute Liver Failure**	73
	How Should Subjects Be Cooled?	73
	To What Temperature Should Patients Be Cooled	74
	Duration of Hypothermia in ALF Patients	74
	Re-Warming Strategy for Hypothermic ALF Patients	74
	Brain Ammonia	77
	Brain Glucose Metabolism	77
	Disruption of Brain Osmotic Balance	78
	Concentration of Amino Acids in the Brain's Extracellular Space	79
	Brain Microglial Activation	79
	Other Factors in the Brain	80
	Systemic Hemodynamics	80
	Systemic Inflammation	81
Chapter 12	**Therapeutic Hypothermia in Ischemic Stroke**	83
	Therapeutic Hypothermia in Experimental Ischemic Stroke	83

	The Effect of Hypothermia on Brain Metabolism..............83
	Hypothermia as a Neuroprotective Strategy: Influencing Cell Death Mechanisms 84
	Hypothermia and Cell Survival Pathways.........................85
	Anti-Inflammatory Impacts of Therapeutic Hypothermia..85
	Optimal Target Temperature 86
	Duration of Cooling...87
	Brain Cooling 88
Chapter 13	**The Implementation of Hypothermia in Traumatic Brain Injury**...91
	Clinical Trials 91
	Experiments Using Hypothermia in TBI..........................94
	The Pathophysiology of Trapeutic Hypothermia in Traumatic Brain Injury...95

Conclusion and Suggestions..97

References 99

About the Authors 103

Index 105

Preface

".... and whoever brings a person to life, it is as if he has brought all mankind to life"
"The Holy Quran, Surah Al-Ma'idah, verse 32"
"In the name of the one who taught mankind to think"

According to the American Heart Association, the primary objective in advanced cardiopulmonary resuscitation is cerebral resuscitation. This focus on brain preservation has led to the widespread adoption of the term "cardiopulmonary and cerebral resuscitation (CPCR)" over "cardiopulmonary resuscitation (CPR)". A key strategy for achieving this goal is the induction of mild hypothermia in patients who have experienced cardiac arrest. Since 2003, the American Heart Association has advocated for this approach for all patients who regain a spontaneous pulse yet remain unconscious following resuscitation, making it a standard requirement starting in 2010. The implementation of mild hypothermia post-resuscitation has significantly decreased mortality rates and enhanced neurological outcomes in these patients compared to those who maintained normal body temperature. The broader application of therapeutic hypothermia has also transformed treatment protocols for individuals with severe brain injuries and comas. Moreover, it plays a crucial role in managing conditions such as strokes, heart attacks, and hepatic encephalopathy, topics that are further explored in this book. In the summer of 2011, during a fellowship at the Vienna University of Medical Sciences, Austria, I witnessed remarkable recoveries. Patients who were unconscious post-cardiac arrest but had a spontaneous pulse responded exceptionally well to a 48-hour hypothermia protocol, often being able to walk out of the hospital. Motivated by the critical importance of cerebral resuscitation and therapeutic hypothermia post-resuscitation, I decided to author a comprehensive book on these topics. It is my hope that this guide will be extensively utilized in emergency and intensive care settings, providing substantial benefits to those in need.

This book is an outcome of my direct experiences with hypothermia treatment in cardiac arrest cases and would not have been feasible without the cooperation and encouragement from many dedicated individuals. To them, I extend my deepest thanks for their invaluable contributions to my educational journey and professional endeavors.

Professor Gunnar Ohlen (Director of the Department of Emergency Medicine, Karolinska University, Stockholm, Sweden and former President of the European Society of Emergency Medicine), and Professor Kambiz Sarahrudi (Honored Faculty Member of the Department of Traumatology, Vienna University of Medical Sciences)

Dr. Tannaz Novinbahador, biochemist at the Immunology Research Center, Tabriz University of Medical Sciences, Tabriz, Iran, and Dr. Farzad Rahmani, Associate Professor of the Department of Emergency Medicine, Tabriz University of Medical Sciences, who have made valuable efforts in compiling the book, and without their efforts, the present collection would certainly not have been possible.

Finally, I deem it my duty to express my profound gratitude and appreciation for the steadfast support of my esteemed wife, Prof. Minou Gharehbaglou, Faculty of Architecture, Tabriz Islamic Art University, Tabriz, Iran, and my beloved daughter, Setia. I extend my best wishes to them from this unique perspective.

Hassan Soleimanpour
Professor of Anesthesiology and Critical Care, Emergency Medicine Department, Tabriz University of Medical Sciences, Tabriz, Iran
Clinical Fellowship in EBM, Joanna Briggs Institute, University of Adelaide, Australia
Fellowship in Trauma Critical Care and CPR, Vienna, Austria
Subspecialty in Intensive Care Medicine (ICM), Tabriz University of Medical Sciences, Tabriz, Iran

Acknowledgments

We would like to thank the Clinical Research Development Unit at Imam Reza General Hospital, Tabriz University of Medical Sciences in Tabriz, Iran, for their cooperation in conducting this research.

Introduction and History

In the general population aged 35 and above, the occurrence of sudden cardiac arrest is roughly 1 in every 1000 individuals. It is projected that fewer than 10% of these individuals, who suffer from severe neurological impairment due to hypoxic brain injury, will achieve full neurological recovery. Annually, Europe experiences about 375,000 instances of sudden cardiac arrest [1]. Out-of-hospital cardiac arrests account for approximately 78,000 of these cases each year, with the survival rate to hospital discharge being around 5%. The primary objective of existing cardiopulmonary resuscitation guidelines and the efforts of emergency physicians is to restore effective cardiac rhythm through the use of defibrillation, chest compressions, and pharmacological interventions. Nonetheless, the prognosis for patients who regain spontaneous circulation after undergoing cardiopulmonary resuscitation remains dismal. Of those who are admitted to the intensive care unit following resuscitation from a cardiac arrest, about 25-40% survive until hospital discharge. Regrettably, the majority of individuals who are successfully resuscitated will need continuous care or will suffer from significant cognitive and memory deficits. The economic and human toll associated with brain injuries due to oxygen deprivation remains unquantified, yet it is believed to be considerable. Accurately determining the total fatalities caused by sudden cardiac arrest proves challenging. Surveys from the United States indicate that each year, over 300,000 individuals succumb to sudden cardiac death, with global estimates potentially reaching into the millions [2]. It is essential to acknowledge Prof. Peter Safar when discussing post-resuscitation hypothermia, as he is widely recognized as its pioneer. Born in Vienna, Austria in 1924, Prof. Peter Safar is often referred to as the father of modern resuscitation techniques. His parents were both medical professionals, his father a surgeon and his mother a pediatrician. After earning his medical degree in oncology from the Medical University of Vienna, he moved to the United States to further his education in anesthesia and went on to publish the inaugural Guidelines for community-wide emergency medical services. He established the International Resuscitation Research Center (IRRC) at the University of Pittsburgh, where he was the director until 1994. Throughout his illustrious career, Prof. Peter Safar was nominated for the Nobel Prize in Medicine three times and authored over 1,300 scientific papers, 600 abstracts, and numerous books and booklets exceeding 30 in total. He was also fervently dedicated to human rights and promoted what he termed the "medicine of peace and friendship." Prof. Peter Safar passed away on August 3, 2003, at the age of 79.

Abbreviations

AST	Aspartate Aminotransferase
ALT	Alanine Aminotransferase
ATP	Adenosine Triphosphate
BBB	Blood-Brain Barrier
BT	Bleeding Time
CPR	Cardiopulmonary Resuscitation
DNR	Do Not Resuscitate
EMS	Emergency Medical Service
ERC	European Resuscitation Council
ICP	Intracranial Pressure
IVC	Inferior Vena Cava
ILCOR	International Liaison Committee on Resuscitation
LVICF	Large Volume of Intravenous Cold Fluid
MAP	Mean Arterial Pressure
PFC	Perfluorocarbon
PEA	Pulseless Electrical Activity
SBP	Systolic Blood Pressure
TOF	Train Of Four
VF	Ventricular Fibrillation
VT	Ventricular Tachycardia
HACA	The Hypothermia After Cardiac Arrest Study
ILCOR	the International Liaison Committee on Resuscitation
ICT	Intracerebral temperature or
r-tPA	recombinant tissue plasminogen activator
TXA2	Endothelin and thromboxane A2
PGE2	Prostaglandin E2
SvcO2	Central venous oxygen saturation
ANP	atrial natriuretic peptide
ADH	antidiuretic hormone
CBT	core body temperature

ICP	intracranial pressure
SOFA	Sequential Organ Failure Assessment
SSD	Therapy Selective Digestive Decontamination
GCS	Glasgow Coma Scale
PNS	peripheral nerve stimulator
ETCO$_2$	end-tidal carbon dioxide
ECMO	Extracorporeal membrane oxygenation
CPB	Cardiopulmonary bypass
ROSC	return of spontaneous circulation
RCTs	Randomized Controlled Trials
CA	Cardiac ARREST
FROST-I	Finding the Optimal Cooling Temperature After Out-of-Hospital Cardiac Arrest
OHCA	Out-of-Hospital Cardiac Arrest
AHA	American Heart Association
CPCR	cardiopulmonary cerebral resuscitation
CPR	cardiopulmonary resuscitation
HACA	hypothermia after cardiac arrest
ROSC	post-return of spontaneous circulation
AMI	Acute myocardial infarction
TH	therapeutic hypothermia
CAO	coronary artery occlusion
PCI	Percutaneous Coronary Intervention
ROS	Reactive oxygen species
ATP	adenosine triphosphate
LADl	eft anterior descending
AAR	area at risk
MI-ICE	Myocardial Infarction - Immediate and Comprehensive Evaluation
MACE	major adverse cardiac events
ERK	Extracellular Signal-Regulated Kinase
mPTP	permeability transition pore
STEMI	ST-Elevation Myocardial Infarction
ALF	Acute liver failure
ICH	Intracerebral Hemorrhage
ICP	Intracranial Pressure
OLT	orthotopic liver transplantation
APAP	N-acetyl-para-aminophenol
CPP	cerebral perfusion pressure

Abbreviations

TNF-α	Tumor Necrosis Factor-alpha
IL-6	Interleukin-6
CBF	Cerebral blood flow
SNAT	Sodium-Coupled Neutral Amino Acid Transporter 5
NOS	nitric oxide synthase
CaSR:	calcium-sensing receptor
GABA-B-R1	gamma-aminobutyric acid B receptor 1
PKC	protein kinase C
RBM3	RNA-binding motif protein 3
BDNFb	rain-derived neurotrophic factor
GNF	glial-derived neurotrophic factor
NT	neurotrophins
ERK1/2	extracellular signal-regulated kinase-1/2
PTEN	phosphatase and tensin homolog
NF-kB	nuclear factor-kB
AK/STAT	Janus kinase/signal transducer and activator of transcription
TGF-b	transforming growth factor beta
mRS	Modified Rankin Scale
TBI	Traumatic brain injury
GCS	Glasgow Coma Scale
BIS	Bispectral Index

Chapter 1

Review of the Literature

The origins of therapeutic hypothermia as a medical treatment trace back to the 1950s. During this period, moderate hypothermia, maintaining body temperatures between 28-32°C, was employed to safeguard the brain during ischemic episodes and surgeries involving the heart and brain. Subsequently, in the 1960s, Prof. Peter Saffer introduced the concept of utilizing moderate hypothermia following cardiac arrest within the cardiopulmonary resuscitation protocols. Over the subsequent 25 years, various complications associated with this approach were identified, including shivering, vasospasm, heightened plasma viscosity and hematocrit levels, reduced blood coagulation, ventricular fibrillation, and diminished infection resistance. Additionally, the challenges of both inducing and sustaining moderate hypothermia in patients proved significant. Consequently, the application of moderate hypothermia in post-cardiac arrest scenarios was phased out. Research focus shifted towards animal studies exploring mild hypothermia, which yielded promising neurological results in models subjected to extended cardiac arrest. During the 1980s, comprehensive studies on canine subjects assessed the effects of mild hypothermia post-cardiac arrest. These investigations involved reducing brain temperature to 34°C after natural circulation restoration using surface cooling techniques on the head and neck, along with peritoneal lavage using chilled Ringer's solution, maintaining this reduced temperature for 12 hours. The findings indicated that dogs experiencing ventricular fibrillation for 10-12 minutes exhibited enhanced neurological functions. Furthermore, no adverse cardiovascular effects were observed in any of the studies concerning mild hypothermia [3].

Concurrently, similar research involving rodents demonstrated that mild hypothermia could enhance neurological outcomes. Following these findings, multiple human clinical trials were initiated to explore the effects of mild hypothermia post-cardiac arrest, particularly focusing on its potential to improve neurological functions and decrease mortality rates [4]. One of the earliest such trials was led by Dr. Lenov Y and his team, involving a multicenter study across Europe that exclusively selected patients exhibiting asystole and pulseless electrical activity. The study involved cooling 30 patients using a Figicap, which applied cold temperatures to the head and neck areas. The cooling was ceased once the patient's body temperature reached 34°C or after four hours, followed by a passive rewarming period over eight hours. Among the 16 patients treated with hypothermia, two showed favorable neurological outcomes. In contrast, none of the non-hypothermic group displayed such improvements. Survival rates showed that three patients from the hypothermic group and one from the control group lived past the trial. Additionally, four patients in the hypothermic group and five in the control group reported reduced urinary output, with no further adverse events noted. In research led by Dr. Bernard S in 2002, involving 77 individuals who experienced cardiac arrest outside of hospital settings, the core body temperature of these patients was reduced to 33°C within two hours following the restoration of spontaneous circulation and was maintained at this level for up to 12 hours. The main goal of this research was to assess the patients' cerebral function at the time of discharge to their homes or a rehabilitation facility. The findings indicated that 49% of the patients in the hypothermic group exhibited favorable neurological outcomes compared to 26% in the control group. The mortality rates were 51% for the hypothermic group and 68% for the control group, with no significant difference in adverse events between the two groups [5]. In another investigation, "The Hypothermia After Cardiac Arrest Study (HACA)" conducted by Dr. Fritz Sterz, included 273 patients who suffered from cardiac arrests outside of hospitals and 10 patients from within hospital settings, primarily during surgical procedures. Here, the core body temperature was elevated to 32-34°C within four hours after spontaneous blood circulation resumed and was sustained at this temperature for up to 24 hours. The primary aim of this study was to evaluate the preservation of good cerebral function six months post-arrest, defined as either normal brain function or sufficient function for independent living and part-time employment. A secondary goal was to assess the incidence of complications within the first seven days post-arrest or death within six months [6]. The findings of the research indicated that 55% of patients in the hypothermic group and 39% of those in the control group exhibited satisfactory neurological outcomes. The death rate was 41% in the hypothermic group, compared to 55% in the control group. Despite facing a greater incidence of complications such as bleeding, pneumonia, and sepsis, these occurrences in hypothermic patients did not significantly differ from those in normothermic patients statistically [7]. Furthermore, a meta-analysis of three clinical trials assessing the effects of mild hypothermia following cardiac arrest revealed that patients in the hypothermic group were more likely to be discharged with favorable neurological recovery. Additionally, a higher survival rate at six months was observed in the hypothermic group compared to the control group. In a study conducted by Bernard and colleagues, 22 individuals who experienced diminished consciousness after a cardiac arrest (with 8 patients initially presenting rhythms other than ventricular fibrillation) underwent mild hypothermia treatment. This was achieved by administering cold (4°C) Ringer lactate intravenously at a dosage of 30 ml per kilogram of body weight. Of these, 10 patients, including 2 whose initial rhythms were not ventricular fibrillation, were successfully discharged from the hospital. Additional research in this area consistently demonstrates the effectiveness of mild hypothermia in patients who achieve spontaneous circulation following a cardiac arrest, particularly those with an initial ventricular fibrillation rhythm and those occurring outside of hospital settings [8]. Mild hypothermia has also shown positive outcomes in other rhythmic disturbances and during in-hospital cardiac arrests.

In 2003, the International Liaison Committee on Resuscitation (ILCOR) issued guidelines recommending that "all patients who are resuscitated from cardiac arrest and regain spontaneous circulation (assuming their initial rhythm was ventricular fibrillation and they remain unconscious) should undergo cooling to 32–34°C for 12–24 hours. The most recent guidelines from the American Heart Association have also integrated a hypothermia protocol for post-cardiac arrest care into their treatment algorithm.

Chapter 2

The Mechanism of Action of Therapeutic Hypothermia

To effectively implement hypothermia in medical practice, a thorough understanding of its action mechanisms and potential adverse effects is crucial. Lack of this knowledge can diminish its therapeutic benefits or even result in treatment failures. Historical accounts from the 1950s and 1960s document significant complications when hypothermia was first applied to treat conditions like cardiac arrest and traumatic brain injury. Initially, it was believed that hypothermia primarily exerted its beneficial effects by decreasing metabolic rates and lowering oxygen and glucose usage in brain cells. However, recent findings suggest that hypothermia also enhances neurological outcomes through various other processes. A key advancement in the application of therapeutic hypothermia is the observation that mild to moderate hypothermia (31-35°C) not only improves neurological outcomes more effectively than severe hypothermia (≤30°C) but also presents fewer side effects. Another significant progress in this field is the expansion of intensive care unit capacities, which facilitates the treatment of patients requiring immediate and sophisticated care. Research indicates that the success of hypothermia treatment hinges on the promptness of the cooling initiation, the duration of the cooling period, the rate at which patients are rewarmed, and effective side effect management. Since different pathophysiological mechanisms can cause varied complications post-cardiac arrest, the timing and length of hypothermia application may need to be tailored to each patient's specific condition. It is essential to recognize that a thorough comprehension of the diverse protective mechanisms afforded by hypothermia can significantly aid in meeting therapeutic objectives and enhancing neurological outcomes for patients, as we will explore further.

Brain Metabolism

Initially, when hypothermia was applied in medical settings, it was believed that its sole beneficial effect was the reduction of brain metabolism. Specifically, for every 1°C reduction in temperature, brain metabolism is lowered by 5-8%. This reduction results in decreased oxygen and glucose usage by brain cells. Nonetheless, this is not the singular benefit of hypothermia; there are additional mechanisms at play that may be equally or more significant.

Apoptosis, Calpain-Related Proteolysis, and Mitochondrial Dysfunction

In scenarios of ischemia/reperfusion following the resuscitation of patients after a cardiac arrest, cells might either undergo necrosis or their functions could be fully or partially restored. These cells might also proceed along the pathway of apoptosis and programmed cell death. Apoptosis is influenced by various cellular processes including mitochondrial dysfunction, disturbances in cellular metabolism, and the release of different enzymes. Research has indicated that hypothermia can disrupt the apoptosis pathway and avert damage that leads to cell death. Hypothermia intervenes early in the apoptosis process, potentially saving cells by inhibiting enzyme activity, preventing mitochondrial dysfunction, curtailing excessive neurotransmitter release, and regulating intracellular ion levels. Given that apoptosis is a detrimental process that can persist for 48-72 hours post-reperfusion, hypothermia plays a crucial role in safeguarding human nerve cells and minimizing damage post-resuscitation.

Ion Pumps and Neuronal Excitation Associated with Cardiac Arrest

Substantial evidence indicates that hypothermia can inhibit the detrimental processes affecting brain cells during ischemia or subsequent reperfusion. In the event of ischemia, the concentration of high-energy metabolites (adenosine triphosphate and phosphocreatine) in brain cells swiftly diminishes following the cessation of oxygen supply, prompting a metabolic shift from aerobic to anaerobic. This shift results in increased levels of inorganic phosphate, lactate, and hydrogen ions within the cells. Consequently, these changes lead to an elevated intracellular calcium level by inducing acidosis both internally and externally in the cell. The depletion of adenosine triphosphate coupled with acidosis hampers the normal cellular mechanisms that expel excess calcium. Concurrently, disturbances in the sodium/potassium pump and the sodium/potassium/calcium channel contribute to a significant accumulation of calcium within the cell. This surge in intracellular calcium impairs mitochondrial function and triggers the activation of various cellular enzymes (kinases and proteases). Alongside these events, the neuronal membrane depolarizes, releasing glutamate—an excitatory neurotransmitter—into the surrounding extracellular space. This release intensifies the stimulation of glutamate receptors on the cell membrane, which under normal circumstances would only briefly interact with glutamate. However, prolonged exposure to glutamate causes hyperexcitation of cells, exacerbating cellular damage. Even after blood flow resumes and glutamate levels normalize, the activation of glutamate receptors continues sporadically, ultimately leading to cell death.

Studies involving the induction of hypothermia in animal models indicate that early application of hypothermia following cardiac arrest can prevent or even reverse neuronal damage caused by excitotoxicity. The timing for initiating hypothermia after the restoration of spontaneous circulation post-cardiac arrest varies, ranging from 30 minutes to 6 hours.

Immune Response

In all forms of brain injury, a pronounced and sustained inflammatory response is triggered within an hour following the ischemia/reperfusion period. High levels of proinflammatory mediators such as tumor necrosis factor-alpha and interleukin-1 are secreted in significant amounts by astrocytes, microglia, and endothelial cells. These levels rise after one hour of reperfusion and stay elevated for up to five days. This inflammatory process stimulates the immune system, leading to leukocytes crossing the blood-brain barrier and accumulating in the brain tissue. Concurrently, the complement system becomes active, resulting in the activation of neutrophils and later, monocytes and macrophages. This often coincides with the generation of free radicals during the reperfusion phase. Certain immune functions, like the phagocytic activity of macrophages, production of toxic metabolites, and stimulation of further immune responses, play crucial roles in exacerbating this cycle of destruction. Research on both animal models and some human studies has demonstrated that hypothermia can reduce these inflammatory responses induced by ischemia and subsequent cytokine release. Moreover, hypothermia helps protect against DNA damage within cell nuclei during reperfusion, lipid peroxidation, nitric oxide synthesis (which is critical in exacerbating brain damage post-ischemia), and leukotriene production.

Fortunately, the initiation of cellular destruction due to immune responses typically starts after more than an hour and takes time to fully develop, allowing a window for hypothermia induction.

Free Radicals

Another harmful mechanism following ischemia/reperfusion is the generation of free radicals, including superoxide, peroxynitrite, hydrogen peroxide, and hydroxyl radicals. These radicals significantly influence whether a cell will undergo apoptosis or recover. The suppression of free radical production correlates directly with the application of hypothermia; as body temperature decreases, so does the production and concentration of free radicals. While hypothermia does not entirely stop free radical production, it substantially mitigates their generation and accumulation, thereby enhancing cellular recovery and function.

Vascular Permeability, Blood-Brain Barrier Damage, and Edema Formation

Ischemia/reperfusion leads to impairment of the blood-brain barrier, resulting in cerebral edema. Treatments like mannitol, used in cases of stroke or traumatic brain injury, may exacerbate damage to the blood-brain barrier [9]. Conversely, hypothermia can protect this barrier by decreasing vascular permeability following ischemia/reperfusion, thereby reducing cerebral edema and lessening the resultant damage. Additionally, hypothermia helps minimize hemoglobin leakage from vessels post-traumatic brain injury. In clinical settings, cerebral edema is assessed by monitoring intracranial pressure. Research indicates that hypothermia lowers intracranial pressure, enhances survival rates, and betters neurological outcomes.

Intracellular and Extracellular Acidosis-Brain Metabolism

During the development of intracellular acidosis, which is crucial in the degenerative process, several factors contribute including damage to cell membranes, malfunctioning of ion pumps within these membranes, mitochondrial impairment, irregular enzyme activities, and disruption of cellular processes. Ischemia/reperfusion also elevates brain lactate levels, which are significantly decreased by employing hypothermia. Furthermore, this condition disrupts glucose utilization in the brain during the ischemia/reperfusion phase. However, studies have shown that hypothermia can improve brain glucose consumption.

Research further suggests that inducing hypothermia during and after the reperfusion phase enhances metabolic recovery. This improvement is facilitated through the preservation of high-energy phosphates such as adenosine triphosphate and by reducing the build-up of harmful metabolites.

Brain Temperature

In individuals with good health, the temperature within the brain (Intracerebral temperature or ICT) can exceed the core body temperature. This disparity in temperature may widen following a nerve injury, with differences ranging from 0.1 to 2°C. Typically, there is no significant variation in temperature across different regions of the brain in a healthy person; however, this can change post-brain injury due to heightened destructive processes in affected areas. It is important to note that an elevation in intracerebral temperature is associated with an increase in intracerebral pressure. Consequently, lowering the brain temperature in patients experiencing cardiac arrest through hypothermia induction leads to reduced intracerebral pressure and subsequently lowers brain metabolism rates. Research has consistently shown that fever acts as an independent factor and predictor for neurological outcomes and mortality in cases of stroke, traumatic brain injury, and anoxic brain injury. While more research is needed to fully understand the link between fever and heightened neurological complications, animal studies have demonstrated that inducing mild hypothermia can prevent fever-related neurological damage and enhance tissue resilience to ischemia.

Coagulative Activity

Research indicates that both cardiopulmonary arrest and subsequent resuscitation efforts are linked to heightened coagulation activity, leading to fibrin deposition and blockages in the microvasculature of the heart and brain. The use of anticoagulants like heparin or recombinant tissue plasminogen activator (r-tPA) has been shown to enhance circulation and survival rates in animal models. Furthermore, thrombolytic therapy may improve the brain's resistance to ischemic conditions. Early interventions with thrombolytic agents during cardiopulmonary resuscitation in cardiac arrest patients have demonstrated potential benefits in extending life and enhancing neurological outcomes. Additionally, hypothermia's influence on reducing platelet count and function, along with altering the coagulation pathway (leading to a minor increase in bleeding risk), may confer a protective effect on both neurological and cardiac functions.

Factors Affecting the Vessels

Regarding vascular factors, evidence suggests that hypothermia impacts the release of endothelial substances such as endothelin, thromboxane A2, and Prostaglandin E2 (PGE2) in the brain and other regions. While endothelin and thromboxane A2 (TXA2) act as vasoconstrictors, Prostaglandin E2 (PGE2) serves as a vasodilator. Thromboxane A2 further promotes platelet aggregation. These elements are crucial for local cerebral blood flow regulation, where maintaining their balance is vital for physiological stability. Post-ischemic disruptions due to brain injuries often lead to an increased production of thromboxane A2, resulting in vasoconstriction, reduced perfusion, and thrombosis in impacted regions. Hypothermia has been observed to potentially rectify this imbalance. Although preliminary findings suggest hypothermia positively influences vascular factor secretion and enhances cerebral blood flow particularly in damaged brain areas, further research is necessary to fully understand this phenomenon. Moreover, local cerebral blood flow is influenced by various factors including

Autoregulation of cerebral blood Flow capabilities, adequate ventilation, blood gas concentrations, and other treatments like mannitol and hypertonic saline.

Ischemic Tolerance

An additional protective benefit of hypothermia is its ability to enhance ischemic tolerance. Research involving animal subjects indicates that lowering body temperature can improve the brain tissue's resistance to ischemic conditions. Consequently, this property of hypothermia has been utilized in various surgical procedures including those related to the vascular system, cardiopulmonary functions, and neurological operations.

Seizure Activity and Other Factors

Non-convulsive seizures are commonly observed in individuals suffering from diverse brain injuries. There is substantial evidence indicating that these seizures can exacerbate brain damage. Research has demonstrated that hypothermia can inhibit seizure activities, suggesting a potential protective role for hypothermia in safeguarding the nervous system.

Chapter 3

The Side Effects of Therapeutic Hypothermia

Hypothermia induces a range of physiological alterations within the body. The activity of most enzymes, which is reliant on temperature, becomes compromised under hypothermic conditions, affecting processes like drug metabolism, blood flow, respiratory functions, and blood clotting mechanisms. While some of these hypothermia-induced changes are physiological, they can be detrimental to patients who are critically ill, necessitating prevention or management. However, not all complications from hypothermia require intervention. For instance, mild hypothermia may cause bradycardia and reduced cardiac output, yet these symptoms typically do not demand specific treatments. Conversely, hypothermia can lead to insulin resistance and diminished insulin production, resulting in elevated glucose levels that must be addressed due to their adverse impact on neurological outcomes in patients.

In the clinical management of hypothermia, the procedure is generally divided into three phases: cooling the patient to the target temperature, maintaining this temperature, and finally rewarming [10]. Each phase presents unique challenges and complications that need medical attention. During the initial cooling phase, before reaching the desired body temperature, patients may experience acute issues such as electrolyte imbalances and disruptions in glucose metabolism, which tend to destabilize their condition and complicate management of these issues. The risk of such complications can be minimized by employing rapid cooling techniques, which include surface cooling combined with the swift administration of chilled intravenous fluids. Once the body temperature is stabilized around 33.5°C, the patient's condition tends to stabilize as well, with reduced risks of fluid loss or shifts in intracellular fluids. At this point, shivering usually ceases or markedly decreases, and there are no significant fluctuations in hemodynamic parameters. This maintenance stage also demands regular adjustments to mechanical ventilation settings and modifications to dosages of vasoactive medications [11].

In the maintenance stage of hypothermia treatment, the likelihood of acute complications, like electrolyte imbalances, diminishes. However, during this period, it is crucial to focus on other potential risks including pneumonia, wound infections, and pressure sores. As the rewarming process begins, there is a movement of electrolytes from the intracellular space to the extracellular space. To mitigate this issue, it is advisable to employ a gradual and controlled warming technique. Rapid warming can potentially reactivate harmful processes. The key complications associated with the induction of hypothermia are explored in further detail subsequently.

Arrhythmia, Hemodynamic Changes, and Cardiovascular Effects

Mild hypothermia, defined as a body temperature between 32-34°C, induces significant alterations in hemodynamic parameters, resulting in reduced cardiac contractility and a lower heart rate (with reductions of approximately 25%). Additionally, this temperature range leads to increased central venous pressure and arterial resistance. As a result of vasoconstriction, there is typically a modest rise in blood pressure (around 10 mm Hg). The impact on cerebral vessels is minimal, thereby maintaining or potentially enhancing cerebral blood flow and metabolic processes, as indicated by the consumption rates of glucose and oxygen. These findings have been substantiated through various research studies involving both adults and children. Hypothermia can also influence the electrocardiogram and cardiac rhythm. The initiation of hypothermia and subsequent decrease in body temperature initially cause sinus tachycardia due to a redistribution of blood from peripheral to central circulation and an augmented venous return [12]. As the temperature falls below 35.5°C, sinus bradycardia sets in, worsening as the temperature continues to drop—for instance, at approximately 32°C, the heart rate may reduce to 40 beats per minute or even lower. This reduction in heart rate stems from diminished diastolic depolarization within the cells of the sinus node. Additionally, alterations in cardiac rhythm manifest as elongated intervals between different waves (P-R, Q-T) and a widening of the ventricular depolarization wave (QRS), occasionally accompanied by Osborn waves.

As previously noted, both diastolic and systolic dysfunctions diminish myocardial contractility, resulting in a 25% reduction in cardiac output. Nonetheless, the decrease in metabolic rate during hypothermia typically matches or exceeds the reduction in cardiac output. Central venous oxygen saturation (SvcO$_2$) often remains stable or may rise due to maintained or enhanced circulatory volume. Bradycardia induced by hypothermia generally does not necessitate intervention. However, if intervention is required, atropine proves ineffective because of the specific bradycardia mechanism associated with hypothermia; alternative approaches such as isoprenaline, temporary rewarming of the patient, or, in extreme cases, transvenous pacing or implantation of a permanent pacemaker may be considered. The likelihood of severe arrhythmias remains low until the core body temperature stays above 30°C. As temperatures drop to approximately 28-30°C, the risk escalates notably, particularly in the presence of electrolyte imbalances. Arrhythmias typically initiate with atrial fibrillation and can progress to ventricular tachycardia or ventricular fibrillation. The hypothermic myocardium is exceedingly sensitive to physical manipulation, increasing the risk of transitioning from atrial fibrillation to ventricular fibrillation. It is important to recognize that the hypothermic myocardium shows resistance to antiarrhythmic medications, emphasizing the necessity to keep the body temperature within a safe range. Enhanced venous return triggers the release of atrial natriuretic peptide (ANP) while decreasing antidiuretic hormone (ADH) levels. This response, along with tubular dysfunction, leads to an increase in urine production, a phenomenon known as "cold diuresis." If not managed, this can result in hypovolemia, renal loss of electrolytes, hemoconcentration, and heightened blood viscosity. The danger of volume depletion becomes particularly acute when patients receive diuretic agents like mannitol for conditions such as traumatic brain injury. An increase in blood viscosity, which rises by 2% for every degree Celsius decrease in core temperature, can obstruct blood flow in smaller vessels. The mechanisms described, together with tubular dysfunction, lead to significant electrolyte shifts and elevated serum sodium and osmolarity levels. Therefore, vigilant monitoring of intravascular volume and fluid balance is crucial in managing a hypothermic patient to prevent and address hypovolemia effectively.

Coronary Blood Flow and Ischemia

Research indicates that hypothermia can heighten the likelihood of a heart attack due to induced narrowing of the coronary arteries. The impact of myocardial ischemia on individuals experiencing hypothermia is contingent upon their existing coronary artery health. While hypothermia can enhance myocardial blood flow in healthy subjects, it may lead to vasoconstriction within atherosclerotic vessels in those with pre-existing coronary artery disease. Evidence from various animal studies and initial human research suggests that early application of hypothermia during treatment could potentially mitigate cardiac damage following cardiac arrest. Consequently, further research is necessary to conclusively determine whether hypothermia indeed minimizes myocardial damage, although current data does not suggest an exacerbation of myocardial damage due to hypothermia.

Electrolyte Disturbances

In patients experiencing hypothermia, disturbances in serum electrolyte levels occur due to enhanced renal excretion of electrolytes and subsequent shifts into cells. This increase in renal excretion can be attributed to alterations in the regulation of circulatory volume, cardiac preload, and renal tubular function. Disturbances in electrolytes, particularly magnesium, are critical as they correlate with negative neurological outcomes. In cases of brain trauma, a lack of magnesium leads to detrimental neurological effects, whereas its supplementation has been shown to diminish secondary cerebral cortex damage and mortality. Magnesium also plays a crucial role in mitigating reperfusion injury and is linked to the constriction of cerebral and coronary vessels [13].

Research indicates that administering magnesium following a myocardial infarction can decrease the extent of the infarct and enhance the function of the remaining heart muscle. Deficiencies in magnesium are also tied to various cardiovascular and respiratory issues including arrhythmias in both ventricles and atria, bronchospasm, seizures, and metabolic disturbances like insulin resistance. Moreover, magnesium imbalances may induce other electrolyte disorders including low levels of potassium, calcium, sodium, and phosphate.

Clinical investigations have identified magnesium deficiency as an independent indicator of poor prognosis in critically ill patients in intensive care units as well as those in general wards. This deficiency is particularly linked to worse outcomes in individuals suffering from unstable angina or myocardial infarction. The administration of magnesium in such scenarios not only lowers mortality rates but also reduces infarct size by promoting coronary vasodilation, exhibiting antiplatelet properties, suppressing cardiac automatisms, and shielding cardiac cells from calcium influx during reperfusion.

Additionally, deficiencies in potassium and phosphate can lead to serious health issues such as arrhythmias, muscle weakness, and neuromuscular complications. Specifically, low phosphate levels weaken respiratory muscles including the diaphragm, heighten the risk of respiratory infections, and prolong the duration of mechanical ventilation dependency. In children, hypophosphatemia can also impair myocardial function and reduce cardiac output. Clinical manifestations of hypokalemia encompass cardiac arrhythmias, muscle weakness, rhabdomyolysis, renal impairment, and heightened blood glucose levels (due to suppressed insulin release). The impact of sodium metabolism imbalances on neurological damage is widely recognized. Both hypernatremia and hyponatremia intensify brain damage. An analysis of the potential complications from electrolyte imbalances indicates that averting hypothermia-induced electrolyte disturbances should be a primary treatment objective in patients suffering from hypothermia. It is crucial to keep magnesium, potassium, and phosphorus levels within or above the normal range for patients with neurological injuries. It is important to acknowledge that serum magnesium measurements might not accurately represent total body magnesium content, as intracellular magnesium can remain significantly low even when serum levels appear normal. In such instances, measuring ionized magnesium provides a more accurate assessment of the body's active magnesium status.

Hyperglycemia

As noted, hypothermia diminishes both insulin sensitivity and pancreatic insulin production. Consequently, individuals undergoing hypothermia treatment are susceptible to developing hyperglycemia, with elevated blood sugar levels linked to higher morbidity and mortality rates. Strict regulation of blood glucose and insulin therapy correlates with decreased morbidity and mortality. Elevated blood sugar levels also increase the likelihood of infections, neuropathy, and renal impairment. Thus, tight control of blood glucose is crucial and vital in hypothermic patients.

Other Metabolic Effects and Blood Gas Levels

Hypothermia triggers an increase in the levels of glycerol, free fatty acids, ketones, and lactate, which can lead to a mild form of metabolic acidosis that typically does not require specific intervention. While extracellular hydrogen concentrations are commonly monitored, it is noted that hypothermia slightly elevates intracellular hydrogen levels. Additionally, a reduction in core body temperature by each degree results in a 5-8% decrease in metabolic rate, which consequently lowers both oxygen consumption and carbon dioxide production. As a result, adjustments to the settings of mechanical ventilation systems are necessary during hypothermia, and blood gas levels should be checked regularly. It is important to consider that blood gas measurements are influenced by the temperature of the blood; blood gas analyzers standardly warm the blood sample to 37°C before analysis. This warming process increases the solubility of gases, leading to elevated apparent pressures of arterial oxygen and carbon dioxide, and artificially higher concentrations of hydrogen ions in the blood.

Coagulation System

Hypothermia leads to a marginal elevation in bleeding propensity due to its impact on several factors including the quantity and functionality of platelets, the synthesis of clotting enzymes, and the inhibitor of tissue plasminogen activator, along with other elements of the coagulation cascade, which collectively prolong bleeding time. Similar to blood gas analyses, routine coagulation tests often yield normal results because the blood is warmed within the testing apparatus. Although hypothermia exerts an anticoagulant effect, this influence is notably minor in patients who are not present with bleeding issues. Research involving individuals with conditions such as traumatic brain injury, subarachnoid hemorrhage (SAH), stroke, and post anoxic coma has not definitively demonstrated an elevated bleeding risk. However, in cases of multi trauma patients experiencing active bleeding, it is crucial to manage and stabilize the bleeding prior to initiating hypothermia treatment.

Infection

Hypothermia impairs immune function and diminishes various inflammatory responses, with its anti-inflammatory properties potentially acting as a safeguard against brain damage. It also reduces the release of proinflammatory cytokines and hinders the movement of leukocytes and phagocytes. Additionally, the insulin resistance and elevated glucose levels associated with hypothermia heighten the susceptibility to infections. Research on hypothermia-related complications indicates that prolonged exposure exceeding 24 hours can lead to a mild to severe escalation in pneumonia cases. Conversely, hypothermia lasting 24 hours or shorter poses minimal to no increased infection risk. Evidence from multiple studies supports the administration of prophylactic antibiotics for gastrointestinal decontamination in intensive care unit patients to lower mortality rates and decrease colonization by resistant gram-negative bacteria. Furthermore, selective decontamination has been found effective in preventing infections during extended periods of hypothermia, suggesting that prophylactic antibiotic use in hypothermic treatment should be considered. Hypothermia's effects on skin vasoconstriction and leukocyte functionality elevate the risk of infections in pressure ulcers, necessitating meticulous attention to prevent such ulcers as their condition typically deteriorates and healing becomes compromised. Additionally, vigilant monitoring is essential for areas with vascular catheters and any surgical incisions.

Furthermore, in hypothermic environments, there is a reduction in the activities of circulating immune cells, as well as diminished recruitment of immune cells and platelets, and attenuated cytokine signaling. Additionally, fundamental immune functions like phagocytosis are compromised. Such weakened responses elevate the susceptibility to infections caused by pathogenic or opportunistic microbes [14].

The Risk of Infection Associated with Therapeutic Hypothermia

Therapeutic hypothermia involves the intentional reduction of core body temperature (CBT) in a medical setting. A meta-analysis that reviewed 23 studies identified clear associations between therapeutic hypothermia and an increase in bloodstream infections, although it did not conclusively link it to a broader risk of infections. This analysis also covered five studies focusing on wound or surgical site infections; however, these studies did not specifically investigate hypothermia as an isolated risk factor. In terms of surgical site infections (SSIs) and wound infections, the occurrence rates were low in both the hypothermic and normothermic groups. Additionally, there was no significant increase in infection rates among the hypothermically treated patients, or the studies lacked the necessary design or power to identify any differences.

In cases of severe head injuries, mild therapeutic hypothermia is applied to decrease intracranial pressure (ICP) and mitigate secondary brain damage. Yet, as with other uses of therapeutic hypothermia, research indicates that this intervention might lead to a higher likelihood of bloodstream infections. A retrospective study looking at 14-day outcomes revealed a notably higher rate of bloodstream infections in patients who underwent mild hypothermia treatment compared to those who received no treatment or were treated with barbiturates under normothermic conditions. Notably, in hypothermic patients who developed bacteremia, Pseudomonas species emerged as the predominant pathogen isolated.

Surgical procedures that are contaminated are often linked to surgical site infections (SSIs), whereas therapeutic hypothermia is associated with an increased risk of bloodstream infections. It is hypothesized that the difference between unintentional perioperative hypothermia and therapeutic hypothermia may be attributed to the demographics of the patient groups involved in therapeutic hypothermia during observational studies: these patients are predominantly non-surgical, thereby eliminating the risk of SSIs, and they are generally in critical condition, which includes having the highest levels of intracranial pressure, placing them at a greater risk for sepsis. The notion that only therapeutic, and not accidental, hypothermia contributes to a higher incidence of bloodstream infections seems improbable. This is supported by a unique study of 6,237 non-surgical patients in the ICU, which showed significantly higher rates of bloodstream infection among those who suffered from unintentional hypothermia, particularly severe cases. Notably, in several studies where an increase in infection risk was observed in hypothermic patients, prophylactic antibiotics were routinely administered. It is believed that the findings discussed here likely underestimate the true escalation in infection risk linked to hypothermia in scenarios where antibiotics are either administered late, not administered at all, or not included in the standard care protocol, such as after a traumatic event in a challenging setting.

In a randomized controlled trial, the application of mild therapeutic hypothermia (32–34°C) to sepsis patients was found to exacerbate respiratory failure, circulatory collapse, and organ dysfunction. These outcomes have been associated with hypotension and vascular dysfunction induced by hypothermia in animal research. Similarly, studies involving patients with severe sepsis or those critically ill from infections have shown increased organ failure in those undergoing hypothermia compared to those maintained at normal body temperature. Patients subjected to hypothermia also displayed a greater incidence of central nervous system dysfunction, shock, and an inability to recover from shock when compared to febrile patients. Aligning with these observations of immune compromise, hypothermia has also been recognized as an independent risk factor for sustained lymphopenia during the initial four days following bacteremia, suggesting impaired immune function and prolonged immunosuppression due to sepsis.

In individuals undergoing colorectal surgery, the occurrence of perioperative hypothermia was found to significantly enhance postoperative vasoconstriction and reduce collagen formation at the site of the surgical wound compared to patients maintained at normal body temperatures who received warming measures. These effects of hypothermia compromise the body's ability to resist infections and delay the process of wound healing. Research involving patients with severe sepsis revealed that those who suffered from hypothermia spent a greater number of days in the ICU and on mechanical ventilation than those who were normothermic or had fevers. Additionally, in septic patients, a positive association was observed between hypothermia and elevated (worse) scores on the Systemic Inflammatory Response Syndrome (SIRS) criteria, whereas fever episodes showed an inverse relationship.

Considering the increased severity of their health status, it is understandable that perioperative hypothermia markedly extends the duration of hospital stays for patients dealing with surgical site infections or severe sepsis. There is a theory suggesting that hypothermia may play an adaptive role during infections in humans, with the higher mortality rates seen in hypothermic sepsis patients possibly reflecting their more critical condition, as indicated by earlier research, rather than a direct worsening effect of hypothermia itself. Supporting this theory, an investigation involving 50 sepsis patients with spontaneous hypothermia who were not actively rewarmed demonstrated a link between hypothermic episodes and timing of death, noting that hypothermia rarely occurred in the last 12 hours before death; indeed, most non-survivors showed increases in core body temperature just prior to death. Nonetheless, the role of hypothermia as a contributing factor to mortality in sepsis remains uncertain. For example, another study focusing on critically ill patients with hypothermia identified it as a mortality risk factor even after adjustments were made for the Sequential Organ Failure Assessment (SOFA) score. Consequently, there is still an ongoing debate about whether spontaneous hypothermia resulting from infection in humans is beneficial or detrimental.

Preventing Infection in Hypothermic Patients

There are effective methods for infection prevention in patients experiencing hypothermia. One method is SDD therapy, an antibiotic prophylaxis that has proven effective in reducing the occurrence of hospital-acquired infections such as bacteremia, colonization by antibiotic-resistant Gram-negative bacteria, and mortality in critically ill patients. It is hypothesized that hypothermia might necessitate the use of prophylactic antibiotics, similar to protocols followed in ICU and surgical settings. Evidence supporting this includes observations that hypothermic ICU patients undergoing SDD therapy faced no greater infection risk than those maintaining normal body temperature. Furthermore, the Global Guidelines for the Prevention of Surgical Site Infection advocate for the pre-surgical administration of 80% oxygen to address the hypoxic conditions at surgical incisions, which can be exacerbated by perioperative hypothermia and elevate the risk of infection; this practice has been found to halve the rate of postoperative wound infections. In addition, research involving animal models indicates that immunomodulators could forestall critical outcomes in septic and hypothermic patients. For example, preventive administration of granulocyte colony-stimulating factor (G-CSF) after mild hypothermia in a rat model of sepsis boosted the levels of circulating leukocytes and neutrophils, thereby enhancing survival rates from 20% to 60%. This suggests that promoting the release of immune cells from the bone marrow may help reduce mortality related to sepsis and hypothermia. Moreover, a study showed that administering intravenous ibuprofen increased core body temperature and significantly lowered 30-day mortality rates in patients with hypothermic sepsis.

Shivering

When the body enters a state of hypothermia, it employs various strategies to retain and generate heat. To minimize heat loss, it enhances sympathetic activity and constricts blood vessels in the skin, while heat production is increased through shivering. Shivering can raise oxygen consumption by approximately 40-100%, which may negatively impact patients with neurological impairments or hypoxic injuries. However, this issue is mitigated in patients who are mechanically ventilated, as shivering does not affect their respiratory efforts. To manage shivering, medical professionals often administer sedatives, anesthetics, narcotics, and muscle relaxants. Typically, low doses of narcotics are effective in controlling shivering. In situations where muscle relaxants or narcotics are not suitable, alternative therapies such as neostigmine, clonidine, and ketanserin may be used, though their potential side effects, such as the exacerbation of hypothermia-induced bradycardia by clonidine, must be carefully considered.

Other Side Effects

Hypothermia significantly influences drug metabolism and pharmacokinetics, primarily through its impact on enzymes that are sensitive to temperature changes. While the specific effects of temperature variations on the metabolism and elimination of many drugs utilized in settings such as intensive care units or emergency departments remain unclear, there is an indication that hypothermia generally decreases the clearance rates of several drugs, including propofol, muscle relaxants, fentanyl, and barbiturates.

Hypothermia induces numerous alterations in laboratory findings, such as:

- Elevated levels of serum amylase
- Slight to moderate reduction in platelet count (ranging from 100,000 to 30,000)
- Raised levels of serum lactate
- Hyperglycemia
- Imbalances in electrolytes, including decreased levels of magnesium, potassium, phosphorus, and calcium
- Increased liver enzymes, specifically aspartate aminotransferase and alanine aminotransferase
- Mild metabolic acidosis
- Minor coagulation abnormalities
- Variations in blood gas measurements

Fortunately, while hypothermia carries its own risks, many of the potential complications associated with inducing hypothermia can be mitigated or managed effectively in an intensive care environment. The approach to treating patients differs based on the severity and length of the hypothermic episode, as well as any pre-existing conditions they may have. Generally, employing hypothermia as a treatment for patients with traumatic brain injuries or strokes is more complex compared to its use in individuals recovering from cardiac arrests and subsequent resuscitation. It is crucial that all healthcare providers, including medical and nursing personnel, understand both the physiological and pathophysiological alterations induced by hypothermia. They should also be able to discern which complications are in need of intervention and which are not.

Chapter 4

Inclusion and Exclusion Criteria for Hypothermia Implementation

Eligibility criteria for inclusion are as follows:

- Patients who have been resuscitated from an initial cardiac rhythm of ventricular tachycardia or ventricular fibrillation, with a witnessed arrest.
- Consideration of pulseless electrical activity of the heart, though more research is needed in this area.
- Achievement of spontaneous circulation within 60 minutes.
- A post-resuscitation Glasgow Coma Scale (GCS) score of 8 or lower.
- Individuals aged between 18 and 75 years.
- Resuscitation initiated within 5 to 15 minutes following cardiac arrest.
- Informed consent obtained.

Criteria for exclusion are categorized into absolute and relative:

Absolute:

- Existence of a "Do not resuscitate" order.
- Pregnancy
- Severe cardiogenic shock, defined as systolic blood pressure below 90 mmHg or mean arterial pressure below 50 mmHg for over 30 minutes, despite vasopressor therapy.
- Core body temperature below 30°C (86°F)
- Cerebral hemorrhage.
- Absence of intubation in patients

Relative:

- Comatose states resulting from factors other than cardiac arrest (e.g., trauma, drug overdose, stroke).
- Potentially fatal arrhythmias.
- Evidence of ischemia on the patient's electrocardiogram.
- QT interval exceeding 470 milliseconds.
- Patients younger than 17 years should be evaluated by a pediatrician.
- More than 6 hours elapsed since the occurrence of cardiac arrest.
- Systemic infections or sepsis.
- Conditions predisposing to bleeding of unknown origin.
- Current use of warfarin; consideration of its antidote is advised.
- Arterial blood oxygen saturation levels below 85%.
- Any condition deemed by the attending physician as a contraindication to treatment.
- Pre-existing coma prior to the cardiac arrest.

Chapter 5

Patient Sedation and Analgesia

In the course of implementing mild hypothermia, it is essential to ensure the patient's comfort and alleviate any pain. To inhibit shivering, which is a common response to hypothermia, several pharmacological agents should be administered. These include opioids, sedatives, and muscle relaxants [15].

Opiates

Meperidine

Meperidine, also known as pethidine, is the preferred opioid for managing patient shivering, available in a dosage form of 1 cc equaling 50 mg. The recommended dosage ranges from 1 to 1.5 mg per kilogram of body weight and is administered intravenously. The drug begins to take effect within 5 minutes, with peak effects occurring between 5 to 10 minutes, and its action lasts for about 2 to 3 hours. Continuous infusion rates for the drug vary from 100 to 400 micrograms per kilogram per hour. However, meperidine is contraindicated in patients taking serotonergic drugs because it can induce serotonin syndrome, thereby worsening the patient's clinical state. The primary metabolite of meperidine is normeperidine, which possesses neurotoxic characteristics and is eliminated via the kidneys. The neurotoxic effects of normeperidine are particularly concerning in individuals with renal impairment or chronic users due to the potential buildup of the metabolite, increasing their risk of seizures. Consequently, meperidine is generally not recommended for these groups. Moreover, its use in pediatric settings is typically avoided.

Morphine

Morphine sulfate is another type of opioid available in a dosage form of 10 mg per 1 cc. Compared to meperidine and fentanyl, morphine triggers a higher release of histamine. Common side effects include nausea and hypotension, which generally do not require special treatment. The initial dose of morphine is 0.1 mg per kg of body weight, with the onset of effects occurring within 1-2 minutes, reaching peak effects between 3-5 minutes, and lasting 1-2 hours when administered intravenously. To maintain analgesia and sedation, the infusion rate should be between 1-5 mg per hour. Morphine-6-glucuronide is its active metabolite. In cases where the patient's hemodynamic status is unstable, fentanyl, which is discussed later, is recommended. Due to its cost-effectiveness, availability, and efficacy, morphine is considered an appropriate sedative medication for patients with stable vital signs.

Fentanyl

Fentanyl is an alternative medication that can be combined with sedatives to alleviate discomfort in patients (it is available in a dosage form of 1 cc = 50 micrograms). This drug triggers less histamine release and has a shorter active period compared to traditional opioids. Fentanyl is significantly more potent than morphine, being 50-100 times stronger, and its starting dose ranges from 1-3 micrograms per kilogram of body weight, administered via intravenous injection. The drug's effects begin in under one minute, reaching peak efficacy between 2-5 minutes post-injection, with the duration of action lasting between 30-60 minutes. To maintain sedation, the infusion rate is set at 2-10 micrograms per kilogram of body weight per hour. Rapid administration or high doses of fentanyl (exceeding 5-15 micrograms per kilogram) may lead to wooden chest syndrome, which causes difficult ventilation in patients [16]. This syndrome can be managed with depolarizing agents, although the use of naloxone in such cases remains a subject of debate.

Remifentanil

Remifentanil is an opioid as effective as fentanyl, characterized by its swift action onset within less than 10 minutes, and is available in reconstitutable powders of 1, 2, and 5 mg to achieve a concentration of 50 micrograms per 1 cc. Unlike many opioids, it is not processed by the liver or kidneys but instead by nonspecific esterases. The infusion dosage ranges from 0.1 to 1.5

micrograms per kilogram of body weight per minute. Its adverse effects are comparable to those of fentanyl, including the potential for causing chest wall rigidity. Alfentanil, a derivative of fentanyl, possesses half the potency and one-third the duration of action compared to fentanyl, yet it acts four times quicker (available in a dosage form of 50 micrograms per 1 cc). It presents fewer cardiovascular side effects than both fentanyl and remifentanil. The recommended infusion rate for alfentanil is 0.5-2 micrograms per kilogram of body weight per hour.

Sufentanil

Sufentanil, a member of the fentanyl family, exhibits a potency that is approximately 2 to 2.5 times that of fentanyl and has an action duration ranging from 30 to 40 minutes, with a dosage formulation of 5 micrograms per 1 cc. A notable advantage of sufentanil over other opioids is its minimal effect on patient hemodynamics. Considering the critical role of administering maintenance doses of opioids during hypothermia following cardiac arrest, the specific dosages are detailed in Table 5.1.

Table 5.1. Maintenance infusion rate of opioids used in hypothermia

Drug Name	Maintenance Infusion Rate
Alfentanil	0.5–2 µg/kg/min
Sufentanil	0.5–1.5 µg/kg/h
Fentanyl	2–10 µg/kg/h
Remifentanil	0.1–1 µg/kg/min
Meperidine	100–400 µg/kg/h
Morphine	5–20 mg/70 kg body weight/4 hours

Sedatives

Midazolam

In this case, the optimal medication is midazolam, available in a dosage form of 1 cc equaling 5 mg. Midazolam, a short-acting benzodiazepine that also acts as a beta-adrenergic receptor agonist, typically has a sedative dose ranging from 0.1 to 5 mg and a maintenance dose between 0.2 and 0.04 mg per kilogram of body weight per hour. Following intravenous administration, peak effects are generally observed within 2-3 minutes. It is important to note that midazolam may induce hypotension in individuals with unstable hemodynamics. Additionally, higher doses of midazolam might lead to respiratory depression and paradoxical agitation in patients.

Propofol

Propofol, a beta-adrenergic receptor agonist, is another sedative utilized in medical settings. It is available in a dosage form of 1% or 10 mg per cc [17]. Typically, the initial dose to induce sedation with propofol is 2 mg/kg of body weight. The ongoing infusion rate required ranges from 1-5 mg/kg body weight per hour. Propofol can lead to respiratory depression and apnea, as well as a decrease in blood pressure due to its negative inotropic and vasodilatory properties. The onset of its action occurs within 30 seconds of administration, with effects lasting approximately 6 minutes. The composition of propofol injectable solution includes soybean oil, glycerol, and egg lecithin, making it unsuitable for individuals with allergies to soy or egg proteins. When dilution is necessary, a 5% dextrose solution in water is recommended. The pharmacokinetics of propofol involve an initial distribution half-life of 1-8 minutes, a slow distribution half-life of 30-70 minutes, and an elimination half-life ranging from 4 to 23.54 hours [18]. Propofol infusion syndrome, although rare and potentially lethal, typically arises from administering doses exceeding 5 mg/kg body weight per hour for more than 48 hours. Initially identified in pediatric cases, this syndrome has also been observed in critically ill and elderly patients. Symptoms of propofol infusion syndrome include cardiomyopathy leading to acute heart failure, metabolic acidosis, skeletal myopathy, hyperkalemia, hepatomegaly, and elevated triglyceride levels [19]. The underlying cause appears to be linked to disruptions in free fatty acid metabolism, specifically the inhibition of free fatty acid entry into mitochondria and defects in the mitochondrial respiratory chain [17]. The initial organ affected by propofol infusion syndrome (PIS) is the liver, characterized by elevated triglyceride levels. Therefore, when using propofol for extended sedation, it is crucial to regularly monitor the patient's serum triglycerides every 4-6 hours. Should there be a rise in triglyceride levels, the administration of propofol ought to be halted. It is important to recognize that patients who are critically ill or receiving inotropic support are particularly vulnerable to this condition, necessitating careful use of propofol in these populations. Additionally, there are several techniques to assess a patient's level of sedation, including the Ramsey sedation score. The classification is as follows:

Level 1: The patient is alert, anxious, and restless
Level 2: The patient is awake, cooperative, and calm.
Level 3: The patient obeys commands.
Level 4: The patient is drowsy and responsive to stimuli.
Level 5: The patient is drowsy and has a slow response to stimuli.
Level 6: The patient is drowsy and unresponsive to stimuli.

In the process of inducing hypothermia in patients, it is optimal to attain a sedation level of 4 [18, 20].

Muscle Relaxants

Pancuronium

Pancuronium serves as a long-acting muscle relaxant classified under non-depolarizing agents. When administered via intravenous injection, its peak effect is reached within 3 minutes, and it maintains its activity for about 45 to 60 minutes. The initial dosing for intubation purposes is set at 0.1 mg/kg of body weight, while the subsequent maintenance doses range from 0.02 to 0.03 mg/kg of body weight. Approximately 80% of Pancuronium is eliminated through the urine. The drug triggers a minimal release of histamine and commonly induces sinus tachycardia, which may or may not be accompanied by elevated blood pressure. These cardiovascular responses are primarily attributed to parasympathetic stimulation of the cardiac vagus nerve and, to some extent, the suppression of catecholamine reuptake by sympathetic nerves.

Atracurium

Atracurium is classified as a medium-duration non-depolarizing neuromuscular blocking agent, administered at an initial dosage of 0.5-0.7 mg/kg body weight for intubation and a subsequent maintenance dose of 0.2 mg/kg. Its peak activity is reached approximately 3 minutes post-administration, with its effects lasting between 20 to 30 minutes. About 10%

of atracurium is eliminated through the urinary system, while the remaining 90% undergoes degradation via a process known as the Hoffmann elimination. This particular reaction is influenced by both temperature and the acidity within the body, accelerating with increases in either parameter. However, lowering the temperature below 34°C has a more pronounced impact on reducing Hoffmann elimination than does decreasing body acidity. One of the byproducts of atracurium breakdown is Laudanosine, a compound that poses risks to the nervous system and may induce seizures. Despite this, plasma levels of Laudanosine typically do not rise significantly even with prolonged use of atracurium. Nevertheless, extended use of this muscle relaxant is generally discouraged due to potential neurotoxic effects. Given that atracurium primarily undergoes the Hoffman phenomenon, it remains a preferred option for patients experiencing renal failure.

Vecuronium

Vecuronium is classified as a non-depolarizing muscle relaxant of intermediate duration, with an advised infusion rate ranging from 0.1 to 0.3 mg/kg/hour. It is characterized by its lack of histamine release and its inability to induce hypotension. The elimination of Vecuronium occurs through both renal and hepatic pathways, which can extend its action in individuals with kidney or liver impairment.

Cisatracurium

Cis-atracurium is an intermediate-duration non-depolarizing neuromuscular blocker with an initial dosing requirement of 0.15 mg/kg body weight for intubation and a subsequent maintenance dose of 0.05 mg/kg body weight. The peak effect of this drug is observed within 3 minutes of administration, and its effective duration post-intubation ranges between 30 to 45 minutes [21]. It is entirely metabolized through the Hoffmann elimination process, and like atracurium, one of its breakdown products is Ladanosine. All safety measures applicable to atracurium are equally relevant for cis-atracurium, although it does not negatively impact the patient's hemodynamic stability.

 A peripheral nerve stimulator (PNS) is employed to assess the necessity for muscle relaxants in a patient. This instrument administers four stimulations at intervals of half a second to a peripheral nerve, like the ulnar nerve, and evaluates the extent of blockage by observing the resulting muscle contractions. A score above zero suggests that not all receptors are bound by skeletal muscle relaxants, indicating a need for administration of a relaxant.

It is also essential to consider factors that intensify the effects of nondepolarizing muscle relaxants when determining the correct dosage of these medications.

1. Antibiotics (aminoglycosides)
2. Magnesium sulfate
3. Local anesthetics (procainamide)
4. Antiarrhythmic drugs (quinidine)
5. Furosemide
6. Liver disease

Chapter 6

Initial Patient Assessment

The precise schedule and methods for initiating hypothermia following a cardiac arrest remain undefined. The commencement of hypothermia should coincide with the initial evaluation and stabilization of the patient, which will be outlined according to their priority in the sections that follow.

Airway and Breathing

Patients who are comatose following cardiac resuscitation require a cuffed endotracheal tube to secure the airway and facilitate mechanical ventilation. Various techniques, including rapid sequence intubation or alternatives like finger intubation and cricothyrotomy, may be employed for intubation. In cases where intubation proves unfeasible, tracheostomy may be considered [22]. Mechanical ventilation should commence with a tidal volume set at 10 ml per kg of body weight and a respiratory rate between 8-10 breaths per minute. It is important to recognize that the body's carbon dioxide production decreases by approximately 30% when the core temperature reaches 33°C. As such, the minute ventilation rate should be adjusted downward in hypothermic patients to avoid the risk of hypocarbia, which can be assessed using capnography or arterial blood gas analysis [23]. To support ventilation and expedite the induction of hypothermia, non-depolarizing muscle relaxants are recommended post-neurological evaluation, along with a sedative like midazolam to inhibit shivering. Capnography, a non-invasive technique, measures the partial pressure of end-tidal carbon dioxide (ETCO2) and reflects changes in carbon dioxide levels with each breath [24]. Historically, the ancient Greeks postulated that a combustion engine-like process occurred within the human body, producing "smoke" with each exhalation; hence, the term "capnography" originates from the Greek word "Capnose," meaning smoke. Oxygenation and ventilation are critical physiological processes that must be evaluated in patients who are intubated. Typically, oxygenation is monitored using a pulse oximeter, whereas capnography delivers detailed insights into ventilation, blood flow to tissues, and metabolic conditions breath by breath. It is well understood that carbon dioxide is generated through glucose metabolism in the body and is transported to the lungs via the bloodstream, where it is then expelled through the alveoli during exhalation. Initially, air from the upper airways is expelled, followed by air from the lower airways. The capnogram provides a continuous reading of the carbon dioxide levels throughout exhalation.

Most capnography systems utilize infrared technology. This method relies on the absorption of infrared light by carbon dioxide molecules at a specific wavelength (4.26 μm), with the degree of light absorption directly correlating to the carbon dioxide concentration in the exhaled breath. In individuals with healthy lung function, regardless of age, the disparity between end-tidal carbon dioxide pressure and arterial carbon dioxide pressure remains relatively constant, typically ranging from 2-5 mm Hg. This variance is attributed to alveolar dead spaces within the lungs that do not contribute to gas exchange. The capnography device not only measures the end-tidal carbon dioxide pressure but also displays its corresponding waveform.

Applications for Capnography Encompass

- Verification of correct endotracheal tube placement.
- Oversight of endotracheal tube position during the transfer of patients.
- Evaluation of cardiopulmonary resuscitation effectiveness.
- Utilization as a measure of successful resuscitation.
- Identification of the reasons behind cardiac arrest.
- Tracking of carbon dioxide levels in the blood in patients with elevated intracranial pressure.
- Assessment and prioritization of individuals affected by bioterrorism incidents.
- Determining the severity and monitoring response to therapy in patients suffering from acute respiratory distress.
- Supervision of patients under anesthesia and sedation during minor procedures.
- Assessment of ventilation sufficiency in patients exhibiting reduced consciousness.
- Analysis of metabolic acidosis.

Furthermore, the American Heart Association's 2010 guidelines stipulate that capnography is essential for monitoring during advanced cardiopulmonary resuscitation processes.

Blood Circulation

Numerous research findings indicate that enhanced blood pressure following a cardiac arrest correlates with better neurological outcomes. Utilizing a substantial amount of chilled intravenous fluid (40 ml/kg body weight at 4°C) not only facilitates hypothermia but also elevates blood pressure, thereby improving cerebral perfusion and enhancing the effectiveness of cerebral resuscitation. Should hypotension (mean arterial blood pressure below 90 mm Hg) continue despite fluid administration, inotropic agents must be employed to maintain the mean arterial blood pressure above 90 mm Hg during the hypothermia initiation process. This practice is so critical that facilities like the Vienna Department of Emergency Medicine routinely administer a low-dose norepinephrine infusion during hypothermia induction to avert any drop in blood pressure, even when initial readings are within normal limits. Should there be any decline in the patient's blood pressure, the dosage of the infusion is promptly increased to sustain the mean arterial blood pressure above 90 mm Hg throughout the hypothermia treatment protocol. While epinephrine is often preferred for its minimal cardiac side effects, noradrenaline serves as an alternative in cases where epinephrine leads to complications. If a patient initially presents with high blood pressure, additional sedatives like propofol should be given, and vasodilators such as urapidil can be considered initially, followed by nitrates as a last resort.

The Steps to Be Taken Before Initiating Hypothermia

Once the patient's condition has been stabilized, the initiation of hypothermia may be considered. Initially, placement of an orogastric tube is necessary, followed by the establishment of an arterial line for the purpose of monitoring invasive arterial blood pressure and facilitating the preparation of blood samples for analysis. An electrocardiogram is essential to check for signs of acute coronary syndrome, and a chest x-ray should be conducted to verify the positioning of the endotracheal tube as well as to identify any pulmonary complications resulting from cardiac arrest, such as aspiration pneumonia and pulmonary edema. Prior to starting hypothermia, a CT scan of the brain is recommended for all patients suspected of experiencing a cerebrovascular event to exclude the presence of intracerebral hemorrhage. The insertion of a central venous catheter is critical for monitoring central venous pressure and for the administration of inotropic medications (it is advised not to use this route for administering cold serum during hypothermia induction due to insufficient research in this area). In cases where thrombolytic therapy might be employed, opting for a femoral vein catheter is advised over those placed in the subclavian or internal jugular veins. Continuous monitoring of the patient's blood glucose levels is crucial, as it enhances recovery rates in both cardiac and neurological functions. Regular assessments of hemoglobin, cardiac enzymes, and electrolytes are also imperative throughout the treatment protocol.

Core Temperature Measurement

Continuous and precise measurement of core body temperature is essential during the initiation and application of hypothermia. The temperatures of the brain, bladder, and rectum exhibit minor variations; hence, bladder temperature monitoring becomes more suitable upon hospital admission. In prehospital settings, tympanic membrane temperature monitoring can be employed, though its precision may diminish, particularly when ice packs are applied to the skin. Alternatively, temperature regulation can be achieved through the use of a pulmonary artery catheter; however, this technique is invasive, costly, and demands considerable time. When rapid hypothermia induction (discussed subsequently) is employed, bladder probes are generally discouraged due to their diminished responsiveness to temperature fluctuations.

Measuring the Depth of Anesthesia: Bispectral Index (BIS)

The Bispectral Index (BIS) is employed to gauge anesthesia depth in patients who have received sedative medications. This index, which supersedes the older Guedel system, is a critical tool in medical technology for assessing anesthesia levels. It has become particularly valuable in managing patients subjected to hypothermia, helping to ensure that anesthetics are administered without exceeding necessary doses, thereby minimizing the risk of side effects from drug overuse. The BIS Index also prevents patients from regaining consciousness during hypothermia. Developed by Aspect Medical Systems in 1994, the BIS Index utilizes algorithmic analysis of a patient's electroencephalogram (EEG) to monitor anesthesia depth. When used alongside other monitoring tools like electromyography, it aids physicians in delivering precise anesthetic dosages. The U.S. Food and Drug Administration (FDA) introduced it as one of the premier systems for anesthesia monitoring. At its core, the BIS Index simplifies the complex data from EEG graphs and curves, representing brain cortex activity, into a straightforward numerical scale from zero to one hundred. This scale accurately indicates the anesthesia depth, with zero corresponding to a state akin to deep coma and one hundred to full alertness and consciousness. During procedures involving hypothermia, it is crucial to maintain the BIS Index between 40 and 60 by carefully controlling the infusion of intravenous anesthetic drugs. This practice ensures both the safety and effectiveness of the anesthesia protocol.

Table 6.1. Base index levels based on patient consciousness levels

Level of Anesthesia	Base Index Amount
Full wakefulness and consciousness	100
Responds to normal sounds	80-100
Responds to loud noises or shaking	60-80
General anesthesia, Does not respond to sound stimulation, ability to be conscious and recall is very low	40-60
Very deep sleep	20-40
Severely weakened electrical activity of the brain	0-20
Smoothing of the electroencephalogram waves	0

Chapter 7

Induction of Therapeutic Hypothermia

A major and critical complication of inducing hypothermia following cardiac arrest is the onset of shivering in patients, which necessitates management through the use of sedatives or muscle relaxants. Various methods are available to reduce body temperature, chosen based on what resources are accessible or the practitioner's expertise.

Types of Cooling Methods

Surface Cooling

The most straightforward approach to cool the body post-cardiac arrest involves putting ice packs on the patient's torso, head and neck. Research indicates that this method results in a gradual reduction of body temperature, specifically, a decrease of 0.9°C per hour as noted in the Bernard study (Australian hypothermia protocol) and 0.3°C per hour in the Fritz-Sterz study (Austrian hypothermia protocol). However, this technique is labor-intensive and demands significant time commitment from medical staff. The decrease in temperature occurs more rapidly when utilizing blankets infused with cold water compared to those filled with cold air. However, the process of cooling using either type of blanket—whether water-filled or air-filled—is gradual. Both methods are practical and secure for facilitating mild hypothermia. With advancements in technology, more sophisticated techniques for reducing body temperature have been developed. The latest system employs large adhesive pads with an integrated water circulation system set to a specific temperature, which are applied to the patient's torso and limbs to cool the body effectively (Arctic Sun, Medivance, Colorado, USA). Although limited data exists on the effectiveness of this device in post-cardiac arrest scenarios, it has proven superior to conventional temperature reduction methods for febrile patients in neurological intensive care units. Additionally, it offers the advantages of being both convenient and non-invasive. Alternative surface cooling methods include the application of air currents and alcohol baths. However, these approaches are labor-intensive and have not been thoroughly evaluated in critical care environments. Immersing a patient in ice water is another technique that results in a swift decrease in body temperature, achieving about 9.7°C per hour, which is faster than many other cooling methods. However, this approach is unsuitable for patients in critical condition. In cases of cardiac arrest where spontaneous circulation has been restored, blood flow resumes to the brain before reaching the trunk and limbs. Consequently, employing a cooling cap can be beneficial. Research on this method indicates that the temperature reduction rate is comparatively slower and generally less effective than alternatives like ice packs or cooling blankets. Nonetheless, in infants, who have proportionally larger heads and open fontanels compared to their bodies, cooling caps tend to be more effective than in adults. Another apparatus, known as the emergency cooling system (EMcools pad, Emergency Medical Cooling System), comprises multiple pads constructed from a blend of water and graphite. These pads feature an inner layer composed of a hydrogel that is compatible with human skin and attaches directly to it, facilitating heat transfer from the body. The rate at which temperature decreases using this system is 2.9°C per hour.

High Volume of Intravenous Cold Fluid

A straightforward and cost-effective approach to induce mild hypothermia involves the rapid administration of large amounts of cold intravenous fluids, specifically normal saline and lactated Ringer's solution, at a rate of 40 cc/kg of 4°C fluid. Despite the common occurrence of myocardial dysfunction following extended cardiac arrest, there is evidence indicating that such rapid infusion of cold intravenous fluids does not lead to pulmonary edema in patients. Recent research has shown that administering 4°C crystalloid solutions at 30 cc/kg over 30 minutes effectively lowers the core body temperature without inducing pulmonary edema, with a cooling rate of 1.6°C per hour. Additionally, this technique slightly elevates blood pressure, which has been associated with enhanced neurological outcomes. The fluid is administered through a peripheral vein using a pressure bag, while infusion into the internal jugular or subclavian veins is not advised currently due to limited safety data regarding its impact on cardiac function. This method represents a simple strategy for cooling patients during CPR in field conditions. Although it has not been tested in human subjects, animal studies indicate its efficacy. A potential drawback of this cooling method during cardiac arrest is that it might diminish the effectiveness of defibrillation. Nonetheless, Boddicker et al. have reviewed and concluded that mild hypothermia actually aids in facilitating defibrillation.

Certain contraindications exist for this technique, notably in individuals with pulmonary edema or chronic renal failure who are undergoing dialysis and are unable to handle large fluid volumes. For these patients, it is advisable to use fluids that are both smaller in volume and cooler in temperature. Presently, this approach is recognized as an effective and straightforward means to reduce body temperature and should be implemented promptly following resuscitation. Research on animal models suggests the necessity for further human studies to explore the impacts of applying this technique during the prehospital stage and throughout CPR. Additionally, alternative cooling strategies, such as superficial or intravascular cooling, might be necessary to manage the patient's temperature following the infusion process.

Intravascular Cooling

Currently, a range of closed-ended intravascular catheters is accessible for initiating and sustaining hypothermia. Typically, these catheters are inserted into the venous system, either in the inferior vena cava or the femoral vein, and feature a circulating mechanism filled with temperature-regulated fluid. This chilled fluid moves through a heat exchanger system within the catheter, effectively lowering the core body temperature to the desired level.

Al-senami et al. explored this technique in individuals who suffered neurological impairments following a cardiac arrest. The procedure involved keeping the core body temperature at 33°C for a duration of 24 hours. This was accomplished by placing a closed-ended catheter in the inferior vena cava, and subsequently, the patients were rewarmed. The study reported no negative events associated with this intervention.

Nevertheless, the utilization of the catheter and heat exchange system is constrained due to their high acquisition costs, limiting their application primarily to hospital settings. Additionally, the insertion of the catheter necessitates the expertise of a trained physician. These factors contribute to delays in the initiation of the hypothermia protocol following the patient's admission to the hospital. Nonetheless, employing this catheter facilitates precise temperature management throughout the cooling and rewarming phases of the protocol.

Cardiopulmonary Bypass and Extracorporeal Membrane Oxygenation

The apparatus includes a substantial intravascular catheter (typically intravenous), a blood pump, and a temperature modulation system that facilitates swift and precise regulation of the body's core temperature. Nonetheless, this technique is costly and necessitates the expertise of a trained physician. Furthermore, complete anticoagulation of the patient is essential prior to device attachment. Consequently, this approach is not frequently employed in emergency departments.

Trans Nasal Cooling Device (RhinoChill)

The apparatus comprises a backpack with a total weight of 12 kg, which includes a single-use nasal catheter, a control module, a 2-liter coolant reservoir, and an oxygen cylinder. A combination of oxygen and coolant is delivered to the patient via a connecting hose, with a 10 cm nasal catheter being inserted into the nasal passages at the base. At the end of this catheter, coolant is expelled into the nasal cavity. Here, the coolant encounters oxygen at the catheter's tip and becomes aerosolized. The nebulizing process facilitates heat absorption from the surrounding tissues, effectively reducing the temperature of the nasal cavity to 2°C. The rate of cooling achieved by this method is approximately 1.3°C per hour. The connecting hose links to the control unit, which regulates the cooling speed. It is also important to highlight that this control system has a safety feature; it automatically shuts off if the pressure within the nasal cavity exceeds 60 cm of water [25].

Pharmacological Techniques

In the majority of patients eligible for hypothermia induction, the necessity to employ additional treatments to manage shivering is often essential. For those who are conscious, sedatives alone typically suffice. While there is no universally accepted optimal drug regimen, the combination of meperidine and buspirone is frequently advocated to suppress shivering. For comatose individuals, a regimen of muscle relaxants combined with sedatives is deemed appropriate. Recent approaches have incorporated the concurrent use of magnesium through infusion to aid in the induction of hypothermia. This method has shown promising results in studies, offering enhanced shivering control and a more rapid reduction in body temperature without significant awareness by the patient.

Looking ahead, neurotensin analogs are being considered as a potential treatment option. Neurotensin, a tridecapeptide with receptors predominantly located in the mammalian central nervous system (including humans and mice), increases during periods of hibernation. It is believed that stimulation of these receptors in the brain by neurotensin may induce hypothermia. Recent advancements have seen the combined use of magnesium administration and infusion to promote hypothermia. Research indicates this method enhances shiver control and accelerates temperature reduction, all while maintaining patient awareness. Looking ahead, neurotensin analogs are being considered for similar applications. Neurotensin, a tridecapeptide androgen, has receptors predominantly located in the mammalian central nervous system, including in humans and mice. Typically elevated during hibernation in mammals, neurotensin is believed to activate these brain receptors, thereby inducing hypothermia. A newly identified neurotensin analog can quickly trigger hypothermia upon intravenous administration, eliminating the need for sedation or anesthesia. Remarkably, once neurotensin is metabolized and cleared from the body after 24 hours, the core body temperature naturally returns to normal levels without external heating. In a study conducted by Katz et al. animals subjected to neurotensin-induced cooling demonstrated superior neurological outcomes compared to those cooled externally. However, the safety of this drug for human use remains to be determined.

Ice-Cold Perfluorocarbon Ventilation

For an extended duration, it has been established that mammals are capable of surviving when immersed in a liquid perfluorocarbon medium enriched with oxygen. Subsequently, the development of ventilation techniques utilizing fluids that transport oxygen has been applied to treat patients experiencing respiratory distress. It has been posited that the proportion of lung surface area relative to the oxygen present in a liquid/lung configuration exceeds that in a gas/lung scenario. Yet, clinical trials have not verified the effectiveness of this approach. Moreover, the gradual introduction of substantial volumes of chilled perfluorocarbon into the lungs of a patient leads to a swift reduction in body temperature while ensuring sufficient oxygenation and ventilation. This technique, however, has been explored exclusively in animal studies [26].

Body Cavity Lavage

A recently identified analog of neurotensin quickly triggers hypothermia when administered intravenously, achieving this effect within minutes and without requiring sedation or anesthesia. Furthermore, once neurotensin is cleared from the organism, the core body temperature naturally rises without external warming. In research conducted by Katz et al. animals subjected to cooling via neurotensin demonstrated superior neurological results compared to those cooled using external methods. However, the safety of this compound for human use has yet to be determined.

Ventilation in a Cooled Perfluorocarbon Environment

For many years, it has been established that mammals are capable of surviving extended durations submerged in a liquid environment enriched with oxygen, specifically perfluorocarbons. Subsequently, the development of ventilation techniques utilizing fluids that transport oxygen was introduced to assist patients experiencing respiratory distress. It has been hypothesized that the proportion of lung surface area relative to the oxygen present in a liquid/lung configuration exceeds that of a gas/lung setup. However, clinical trials have yet to verify the efficacy of this approach. Nonetheless, administering large volumes of chilled perfluorocarbon slowly into the lungs of a patient leads to a swift reduction in body temperature while ensuring sufficient oxygenation and ventilation. To date, this technique has been explored exclusively in animal studies.

Lavage of Body Cavities

Numerous research efforts have focused on the impact of using cold fluids to irrigate various body cavities, including the stomach, bladder, and peritoneum. Plattner and his team evaluated multiple cooling strategies alongside superficial cooling methods in a study involving human volunteers. Their comparisons included gastric lavage, involving the infusion of 500 cc of cold fluid every 10 minutes, and bladder lavage, where 300 cc of cold Ringer's solution was administered at the same interval. The initial volunteer experienced abdominal cramps and diarrhea after undergoing gastric lavage, leading to the discontinuation of this approach in further trials. However, bladder lavage led to a reduction in temperature by 0.8°C per hour. Although promising, this technique demands careful implementation and additional nursing staff to manage the fluid exchange. Peritoneal lavage has also been explored, as detailed by Xiao and colleagues. This procedure entails the slow introduction of 2 liters of Ringer's solution at 10°C into the peritoneal cavity, which is then drained after five minutes. The cooling rates observed in the tympanic membrane and pulmonary artery were approximately 0.3°C/h and 0.8°C/h, respectively. While primarily documented for warming patients with accidental hypothermia in emergency settings, its application for cooling post-cardiac arrest patients remains underexplored.

Brain Cooling Alone

To mitigate the adverse impacts of hypothermia, selective cooling of the brain is considered more advantageous. Mori and colleagues have explored the approach of accessing the carotid arteries to introduce chilled blood directly into the brain's circulatory system. While this technique avoids the systemic effects associated with full-body hypothermia, the risks linked to puncturing the carotid artery in emergency scenarios make this method impractical for near-term application.

Time to Start Cooling

Initiation of treatment should occur promptly following the restoration of spontaneous circulation. It appears that a commencement delay of 4-6 hours can still yield a substantial success rate.

Rate and Duration of Cooling

The objective is to reach a target temperature of 33°C within two hours following the return of spontaneous circulation (ROSC) and to sustain this temperature for 12 hours, as per the Australian protocol. Alternatively, the Austrian protocol aims for a temperature range of 32-34°C to be attained within four hours post-ROSC and maintained for 24 hours.

Maintenance of Hypothermia

The length of time for which hypothermia should be maintained following a cardiac arrest remains uncertain. In the research conducted by Bernard, the duration was set at 12 hours, while in the study by Fritz Sterz, it extended to 24 hours. It is crucial to rigorously monitor and manage the core body temperature throughout the treatment period. Reaching a core body temperature of 33°C can induce shivering in adults. While increasing the core body temperature can help manage shivering, this approach contradicts the objective of inducing hypothermia as elevating the temperature above 33.5°C can heighten the brain's demand for oxygen. Consequently, alternative shivering control strategies, such as administering sedatives and muscle relaxants, are preferable over increasing the temperature. Conversely, if the body temperature falls below 32.5°C, it is vital to mitigate the risks associated with moderate hypothermia by removing ice packs, stopping analgesics, and applying a warm blanket if needed.

Targeted Temperature Management

Administering targeted temperature management within the broad range of 32°C to 36°C has historically been a principal approach in enhancing neurological outcomes following resuscitation. This practice was predominantly supported by two minor randomized studies conducted two decades ago. However, recent findings from the TTM2 trial, which involved 1861 participants, have called this method into question. The study revealed that lowering the body temperature to 33°C did not show any advantages over maintaining normothermia at temperatures between 36°C and 37.5°C while preventing fever. Additionally, lower temperature management was linked to higher risks of adverse effects without showing any positive outcomes in the TTM2 trial, suggesting that updating the guidelines to favor normothermia might be warranted.

Contraindications for Targeted Temperature Management

There are limited contraindications for using therapeutic hypothermia in critically ill patients, primarily arising from the exclusion criteria used in earlier randomized controlled trials concerning temperature management. Typically, inducing mild hypothermia is not advisable for alert patients (Glasgow Coma Scale >8), or those with active bleeding, particularly if there is intracranial hemorrhage, as reduced core temperatures could exacerbate these conditions. Conditions such as cardiac arrest due to trauma, sepsis, or hemorrhagic shock are also viewed as contraindications. Managing anticoagulation during hypothermia poses significant challenges; thus, existing coagulopathies are considered a relative contraindication. Moreover, hypothermia can worsen hypotension, making it unsuitable for hemodynamically unstable patients. The feasibility of temperature management in patients experiencing the most severe stage E cardiogenic shock (as classified by the Society for Cardiovascular Angiography and Interventions) and receiving temporary circulatory support like extracorporeal life support remains uncertain. These individuals are at high risk of significant bleeding issues, such as access site bleeding due to severe consumptive coagulopathy and thrombocytopenia. The TTM1 trial indicated no additional neuroprotective benefits when managing temperature at a lower target of 33 °C compared to a milder target of 36°C. The question of whether more precise temperature settings could lead to better outcomes was explored in the FROST-I trial by Lopez-de-Sa et al in 2018. In this study, 150 survivors of out-of-hospital cardiac arrest with shockable initial rhythms were divided into three groups, each targeted to different hypothermia levels—32°C, 33°C, and 34°C—for 24 hours using an intravascular cooling device placed in the femoral vein. The results showed similar favorable neurological outcomes, defined as a modified Rankin Scale score of ≤3 at 90 days, across the groups: 63.3% at 32°C, 68.2% at 33°C, and 65.1% at 34°C. The rates of all-cause mortality at 90 days were also comparable among the groups: 30.8%, 26.5%, and 28.5%, respectively [27].

Temperature Control After In-Hospital Cardiac Arrest

In line with the 2022 guidelines issued by the International Liaison Committee on Resuscitation, alongside recent directives from the European Resuscitation Council and the European Society of Intensive Care Medicine, it is recommended that adults rendered unconscious due to cardiac arrest should undergo fever-preventive temperature management. Currently, the debate continues regarding the ideal target temperature for such interventions. Historically, setting a hypothermic target between 32° and 36°C has been the sole neuroprotective strategy endorsed by international guidelines. Research involving two randomized clinical trials that examined unconscious patients post-out-of-hospital cardiac arrest (OHCA) assessed the benefits of mild therapeutic hypothermia (targeting 32°–34°C) against standard care. These studies demonstrated a notable enhancement in favorable functional outcomes. However, later studies did not replicate these benefits, showing no advantage of hypothermic temperature control over other methods. Predominantly, research on temperature management has been conducted in the context of OHCA. A notable study by Wolfrum et al. which was a multicenter, randomized controlled trial carried out across 11 German hospitals, involved 249 patients who were either subjected to hypothermic temperature control (32-34°C) for 24 hours or maintained at normothermia following in-hospital cardiac arrest (IHCA). The findings indicated no significant differences in survival rates or functional outcomes at 180 days between the two groups. The Hypothermia After Cardiac Arrest in-hospital (HACA) trial similarly found that the differences between hypothermic temperature control and normothermia were not statistically significant, suggesting that the study might have been underpowered to detect meaningful clinical differences [28].

Targeted temperature management (TTM) remains a prevalent approach for improving survival and functional outcomes in OHCA cases. Nevertheless, empirical evidence supporting the efficacy of specific TTM temperatures remains scant. A subsequent study by Doerning et al. in 2025 investigated the relationship between TTM and survival without neurological impairment in non-traumatic OHCA cases across institutions with varying TTM temperature protocols. This study concluded that there was no significant link between a TTM goal temperature of 33 °C compared to 36 °C and survival without neurological damage [29].

Furthermore, an analysis up until 2022 involving one randomized controlled trial and four retrospective cohort studies focused on hospital and

ICU mortality rates showed no significant differences in outcomes between the normothermia and hypothermia groups [30].

Chapter 8

Patient Rewarming Protocol

The initiation of rewarming in a patient, whether following the Australian or Austrian guidelines for hypothermia management, should commence either 12 or 24 hours after cooling begins, respectively. Rewarming can be conducted through passive or active methods. The passive approach involves discontinuing the use of cooling agents such as ice packs or cold serum, allowing the patient's body temperature to rise naturally. Conversely, the active approach necessitates the use of external or intravascular heating techniques to elevate the core body temperature. Research involving animals indicates that the temperature should be raised gradually during this phase. It is also advisable to manage any shivering in the patient with sedatives at this time. Furthermore, as rewarming can lead to peripheral vasodilation, it may be necessary to administer warm intravenous fluids to help sustain normal blood pressure levels.

Patient Rewarming Guide

The increase in temperature should be kept below 0.25°C (0.5°F) per hour, aiming for a core body temperature between 36.5°C and 37°C (97.7°F and 98.6°F) within 48 hours Once the core body temperature surpasses 36°C (96.8°F), sedation should be halted, and then adjusted according to a four-point scale. It is important to note that shivering may persist until the temperature stabilizes at or above 36°C, at which point sedation should be ceased.

Summary

Following the resuscitation of a patient from an out-of-hospital cardiac arrest, current evidence-based medical practices recommend maintaining mild hypothermia in comatose patients to enhance neurological outcomes. The induction of hypothermia involves the administration of a substantial dose of long-acting muscle relaxants and the rapid infusion of cold crystalloid fluids (such as normal saline or Ringer's lactate) at a flow rate exceeding 100 cc/min and a total volume of 40 cc/kg of body weight. It is important to recognize that this method seldom leads to pulmonary edema.

In the protocol for hypothermia, it is necessary to begin and maintain superficial cooling of the patient while monitoring the core body temperature using designated probes located in the pulmonary artery, bladder, and tympanic membrane. The hypothermia treatment should be sustained for a duration of 12-24 hours, followed by a rewarming process that should also occur within 12-24 hours from the initiation of cooling. Presently, initiating hypothermia through extra-membranous systems or solely through brain cooling is impractical due to high costs and procedural complexities. Research indicates that contemporary sophisticated techniques do not offer significant benefits compared to earlier methods.

Chapter 9

The Implementation of Hypothermia in Cardiac Arrest

Pathophysiology of Neuronal Injury in Cardiac Arrest

In the case of cardiac arrest, resuscitation leads to ischemia and reperfusion, which in turn causes nerve damage. Ischemia and hypoxia result in damage to the cell membrane as a consequence of decreased adenosine triphosphate production, impairing the function of the sodium/potassium pump [31]. Additionally, there is an activation of phospholipases that facilitates the degradation of lipids and the release of glutamate, arachidonic acid and harmful neurotransmitters. These processes collectively contribute to an elevation in intracellular calcium levels.

Following the restoration of blood flow after a cardiac arrest, neuronal cells experience a phase of delayed mortality. This process is initiated by the activation of leukocytes due to injury to the vascular endothelium and brain tissue. This injury triggers the release of cytokines and adhesion molecules, which in turn prompts the discharge of oxygen free radicals, proteases, and various cytokines including tumor necrosis factor-alpha, interleukins 8, 6, 1, and 10. These substances contribute to increased vascular permeability, damage to the blood-brain barrier, and the development of cerebral edema. The presence of cerebral edema further complicates matters by extending the distance required for oxygen diffusion and reducing cerebral perfusion pressure, thereby intensifying hypoxia.

The occurrence of sudden cardiac arrest outside of hospitals in industrialized nations ranges from 0.04% to 0.19% annually. When resuscitation efforts are made, between 14% and 40% of these patients experience a return of spontaneous circulation and are subsequently hospitalized. However, only 7% to 30% of those admitted are eventually discharged with favorable neurological outcomes. Achieving positive neurological results following a cardiac arrest is challenging. The actions taken during the resuscitation process and the treatments administered in the initial hours post-arrest are crucial. There is experimental evidence indicating that therapeutic hypothermia may provide benefits in such cases [32].

According to American Heart Association (AHA) recommendations, cerebral resuscitation is the primary goal in advanced cardiopulmonary cerebral resuscitation (CPCR) has evolved significantly since the concept of basic cardiopulmonary resuscitation (CPR) was expanded to include brain preservation in cardiac arrest cases [13]. A critical strategy for achieving effective cerebral resuscitation involves inducing mild hypothermia in individuals experiencing cardiac arrest, a protocol known as hypothermia after cardiac arrest (HACA). In 2003, the American Heart Association (AHA) endorsed the application of HACA for all unconscious adult patients who regain spontaneous circulation (ROSC) following CPCR, specifically when the initial cardiac rhythm is ventricular fibrillation. Furthermore, starting from 2010, it became compulsory to apply this vital protocol universally. The prospects for both short-term and long-term survival, as well as the overall improvement in patient outcomes post-CPR, are greatly influenced by the swift initiation of CPR and subsequent advanced cardiac procedures [33]. In the research titled "The Hypothermia After Cardiac Arrest (HACA)," a total of 283 patients, including 273 who experienced cardiac arrests outside of hospital settings and ten surgical patients within hospitals, were studied. Their core body temperatures were lowered to either 34°C or 32°C within four hours following the return of spontaneous circulation (ROSC) and maintained for 24 hours as per the European/Austrian protocol. The main goal of the study was to assess the restoration of adequate brain function post-cardiac arrest, defined as either normal brain activity or sufficient cognitive ability to live independently and engage in part-time employment. Additionally, the study aimed to track the occurrence of any complications over seven days or deaths within six months post-arrest. The findings revealed that 55% of participants in the HACA group exhibited favorable neurological outcomes compared to 39% in the non-HACA control group. The hypothermia groups mortality rate was 41% and the control group was 55%. Despite a higher risk of complications such as pneumonia, bleeding and sepsis among the hypothermic patients, these differences did not reach statistical significance. Subsequent investigations have explored the application of HACA in various scenarios. Positive outcomes have been observed in stroke patients potentially due to reduced brain swelling and lower intracranial pressure. HACA has also been applied in pediatric cases; however, challenges such as myocardial depression during the induction phase and severe complications during rewarming have led some studies to advise against its use in pediatric cardiac arrests. Conversely, other research has shown improved survival rates in children treated with

HACA, highlighting the need for further investigation in this area. Given the advantages observed with HACA in cases of out-of-hospital cardiac arrests, it is currently recommended after myocardial infarctions, though additional confirmatory research is needed. In one instance involving a 28-year-old patient, HACA treatment yielded positive outcomes.

Pathophysiology of Neuronal Damage in Cardiac Arrest

Neuronal damage can occur during cardiac arrest, following ischemia, or post-return of spontaneous circulation (ROSC). Ischemia and hypoxia result in the cessation of ATP production, malfunction of the Na+/K+ pump, breakdown of cellular membranes, and activation of phospholipase, which triggers lipolysis, the release of arachidonic acid, glutamate, and other harmful neurotransmitters, and a rise in intracellular calcium. Following ROSC, there may be a delayed death of neurons as damage to endothelial cells in arteries and brain tissue leads to the activation of leukocytes and subsequent release of cytokines and adhesion molecules. These events promote the release of free radicals, an increase in vascular permeability, proteases, tumor necrosis factor alpha, and interleukins (IL-1, IL-6, IL-8, and IL-10), compromise of the blood-brain barrier, and cerebral edema. The brain swelling further contributes to unequal oxygen diffusion and reduced cerebral perfusion pressure, perpetuating hypoxia.

Mechanism of Hypothermia

To effectively utilize hypothermia in medical settings, comprehending its mechanisms and potential adverse effects is crucial. Previously, it was believed that the therapeutic benefits of hypothermia were solely due to its ability to decelerate metabolism and lessen the consumption of oxygen and glucose by brain cells. However, current understanding suggests that the positive impact of hypothermia on neurological outcomes also involves additional diverse mechanisms. Research indicates that the outcomes of Hypothermia After Cardiac Arrest (HACA) are influenced by factors such as the rapidity of the cooling onset, the length of the cooling period, the rate at which patients are rewarmed, and the prevention of associated complications. The specific timing for initiating hypothermia and the duration for which it should be maintained vary based on individual patient conditions due to different pathological processes triggered by cardiac arrest. In the HACA protocol, hypothermia treatment typically involves three phases: the initiation of cooling, temperature maintenance, and gradual rewarming, each accompanied by unique challenges that necessitate specific management strategies.

Cooling of the Body Surface

The most basic method for managing Hyperthermia Associated with Cardiac Arrest (HACA) involves applying ice packs to the patient's head, neck, and body. An alternative apparatus is the EMcools pad (Emergency Medical Cooling System), which consists of multiple pads crafted from a blend of graphite and water. These pads feature an inner layer made of hydrogel that is compatible with human skin, allowing for direct contact and efficient heat transfer from the patient. This technique facilitates a heat loss rate of approximately 2.9°C per hour [13, 34].

When Should Cooling Be Initiated?

A recent randomized controlled trial explored the effects of paramedic-led cooling in patients who achieved spontaneous circulation after experiencing a ventricular fibrillation cardiac arrest. In this study, the experimental group was administered 2 liters of ice-cold Ringer's solution by paramedics, whereas the control group began cooling upon hospital arrival using the same technique. The findings showed no significant differences in neurological outcomes between the groups. However, the study did note several limitations, including initial differences in body temperature upon hospital admission. Despite these differences, temperatures equalized between the two groups after 30 minutes and, after one hour, temperatures in the paramedic-treated group exceeded those recorded at hospital entry. In a separate case series focusing on intravascular cooling, the time to reach the coldest body temperature was found to be a critical independent factor for favorable neurological outcomes, with an odds ratio of 0.72 for each hour delay. Conversely, a registry-based case series involving 986 comatose patients post-cardiac arrest showed that the timing of cooling initiation—

averaging 90 minutes with an interquartile range of 60–165 minutes—did not correlate with improved neurological outcomes after discharge.

Potential Risks Associated with Cooling Methods

The adverse effects of therapeutic hypothermia following out-of-hospital cardiac arrest (OHCA) were examined in a comprehensive study involving 22 hospitals across Europe and the United States. This observational, registry-based study lacked a control group, complicating the determination of whether observed complications stemmed from the hypothermia treatment or the cardiac arrest itself. Common complications included arrhythmias (7–14%), pneumonia (48%), and metabolic and electrolyte imbalances (5–37%). However, only sustained hyperglycemia and seizures requiring anticonvulsants were linked to increased mortality. Less frequently observed were sepsis (4%) and bleeding (6%), though these occurred more often with the use of any intravascular device, including angiography equipment, cooling devices, intra-aortic balloon pumps, yet these were not tied to higher mortality rates [35].

A separate report on 11 patients suffering traumatic brain injuries who underwent cooling via an intravascular device for three to eight days showed a deep vein thrombosis rate of 50%. Notably, this rate decreased from 75% to 33.3% when the device was removed within five days in the last five patients studied. Shivering, particularly during the initial phase of hypothermia, is common and can be detrimental as it raises the metabolic rate and oxygen consumption, potentially increasing the risk of myocardial infarction. In clinical settings, however, shivering is typically managed by sedation and sometimes paralysis, which decreases heart rate and raises systemic vascular resistance, ultimately reducing cardiac output. Hypothermia is also associated with various arrhythmias, with bradycardia being most prevalent. While some studies have reported an increase in arrhythmias with hypothermia compared to controls, others have found no significant difference. Additional complications from hypothermia include diuresis-induced hypovolemia that may lead to hemodynamic instability, along with disturbances in phosphorus, potassium, magnesium, and calcium levels. Furthermore, hypothermia impairs insulin sensitivity and secretion, contributing to hyperglycemia and affects drug metabolism, notably leading to a 30% reduction in the clearance of sedative and neuromuscular medications at a body temperature of 34°C [36].

Large Volume of Intravenous Cold Fluids

Administering a substantial amount of chilled intravenous fluids, specifically normal saline and Ringer's lactate at 4°C (40 mL/kg), represents a straightforward and cost-effective method for achieving mild hypothermia. This approach is particularly useful for cooling patients during cardiopulmonary resuscitation in prehospital environments. While this technique has not been tested on human subjects, animal studies have demonstrated its potential effectiveness.

Intravascular Cooling

Various models of closed-end intravascular catheters are presently used for the initiation and maintenance of hypothermia. Typically, these catheters are inserted into the venous system, either in the femoral vein or the inferior vena cava, and feature a temperature-regulated fluid circulation system. Through a pump-connected heat exchanger, cooled fluid is conveyed into the catheter, circulating within it to lower the core body temperature to the desired level [13].

Chapter 10

Therapeutic Hypothermia in Myocardial Infraction

Acute myocardial infarction (AMI) stands as a primary cause of mortality, imposing significant financial burdens on both governments and individuals in countries at all stages of development. The medical community has concentrated efforts on prompt reperfusion therapy and minimizing the size of the infarction to lessen death and disease rates. However, lethal reperfusion injury, which occurs when blood flow is reintroduced to ischemic heart tissue, can lead to the death of cardiac cells and enlarge the infarct area, potentially contributing to 25% of the total damage. Efforts to mitigate reperfusion injury have thus far been unsuccessful, with no effective strategies currently available. Consequently, there is a pressing need for innovative approaches that complement optimal reperfusion therapy to enhance AMI clinical outcomes.

Therapeutic hypothermia (TH) has shown promise in enhancing neurological outcomes for survivors of cardiac arrests occurring outside of hospitals. Implementing TH slowly and even up to 8 hours after spontaneous circulation returns has been associated with increased survival rates and positive neurological results. In the context of AMI, pre-reperfusion application of TH has experimentally shown to reduce infarct size. A core body temperature below 35°C is critical but can be therapeutically achieved under specific medical circumstances. TH is categorized by target body temperatures into mild (32–35°C), moderate (28–32°C), severe (20–28°C), or profound (<20°C). Research indicates a strong link between the target temperature and infarct size reduction; a decrease of 1°C can reduce infarct size by 10–20% in swine and sheep models, suggesting that lower temperatures are more effective. However, temperatures below 30°C often led to atrial fibrillation, and temperatures below 28°C typically induce ventricular fibrillation in most mammals. Mild hypothermia can lower heart rate without impacting stroke volume and mean arterial pressure, and it is typically well tolerated in both experimental animals and humans. A target temperature range of 32–34°C is widely recognized as the optimal goal for TH application.

Critical Period for Hypothermia Management

Delayed and gradual therapeutic hypothermia up to 8 hours after return of spontaneous circulation (ROSC) has demonstrated improved neurological outcomes and reduced mortality in patients who experienced cardiac arrest outside of hospital settings. Conversely, rapid initiation of TH before revascularization is crucial for minimizing infarct size in conscious patients with acute myocardial infarction (AMI). Experimental research consistently indicates that quicker and earlier commencement of TH is more effective at reducing infarct size. Although not always practical in clinical environments, initiating TH even before coronary artery occlusion (CAO) has been shown to achieve maximal reduction in infarct size. Pre-perfusion TH in ischemic models has resulted in approximately 40% reduction in infarct size, although results vary across studies. Therefore, starting TH prior to reperfusion is recognized as a critical strategy. However, initiating TH during reperfusion has not shown a statistically significant reduction in infarct size but has helped limit the no-reflow phenomenon by enhancing microvascular resistance, a key predictor of clinical outcomes in AMI patients.

Types of Hypothermia Induction after MI

Various experimental approaches have been employed to induce hypothermia in AMI models, including surface cooling, endovascular cooling, infusion of cold saline into the coronary artery, extracorporeal blood cooling, peritoneal lavage, total liquid ventilation, and pericardial perfusion. Some of these techniques have been deemed relatively safe and have been implemented in patients experiencing cardiac arrest or myocardial infarction.

A preliminary study introduced a topical pad-type cooling device designed to cover the trunk of patients with acute myocardial infarction (AMI) undergoing primary percutaneous coronary intervention (PCI). This device was confirmed to be safe, although it demonstrated a slow cooling rate of 79 minutes to reach temperatures below 34.5°C, equivalent to a rate of 1.5°C per hour. Trans nasal evaporative cooling involves the administration of a coolant-oxygen mixture sprayed into the nasal passages and brain. This method is portable, straightforward to use, and generally safe but may cause significant nosebleeds in patients with bleeding disorders [37].

Intravenous infusion of cold saline at 4°C initially induces rapid cooling within the first hour due to the infusion of a large volume. However, this technique may lead to respiratory complications from fluid overload and a decrease in cardiac output. An endovascular cooling catheter utilizes a heat-exchange mechanism with a balloon at its tip, which is inserted into the inferior vena cava via a femoral vein. The primary mechanism involves heat exchange through a chilled balloon, avoiding the need for cold saline infusion. Despite the rapid cooling observed in initial studies, broader registry data did not demonstrate such efficiency. Relying solely on the endovascular catheter may not adequately lower the temperature before reperfusion in acute myocardial infarction cases without postponing percutaneous coronary intervention. Recent clinical trials that combined endovascular cooling with intravenous cold saline reported an enhanced cooling rate of approximately 6°C per hour. Automated peritoneal lavage can quickly reach target temperatures owing to its extensive surface area contact, yet it remains an invasive technique. Large-volume peritoneal lavage might cause respiratory distress by elevating the diaphragm and poses risks of significant organ damage from peritoneal puncture, particularly limiting its use in patients with abdominal conditions or severe obesity [38].

Impact of Therapeutic Hypothermia on Infarct Reduction

In cases of mild hypothermia, there is a noted decrease in heart rate while cardiac contractility remains intact, effectively reducing the workload on the heart and its oxygen needs. Furthermore, the overall metabolic rate of the body and heart decreases, leading to a lower demand for oxygen. This reduction in cellular metabolism helps in maintaining adenosine triphosphate (ATP) levels, decreasing the production of reactive oxygen species (ROS), and controlling apoptosis, all contributing to energy conservation and a smaller infarct size. The preventative benefits of hypothermia against ischemia/reperfusion (I/R) injury are also linked to changes in mitochondrial permeability transition pore behavior, diminished calcium overload during cooling periods, and adjustments in cellular signaling mechanisms such as Akt pathways, heat-shock proteins, and extracellular-regulated kinase, which collectively diminish inflammatory responses.

In the context of acute myocardial infarction, particularly with obstructions in the left anterior descending (LAD) artery, therapeutic mild hypothermia has shown promising results in reducing myocardial infarct size and microvascular dysfunction in animal studies. This is especially true when hypothermia is applied prior to reperfusion rather than afterwards. Research by Duncker et al. highlighted a direct relationship between smaller infarct sizes and lower temperatures. Conversely, Maeng et al. observed no advantages when hypothermia was induced during or after reperfusion. Studies achieving target temperatures post-perfusion indicated fewer protective effects when cooling began simultaneously with rapid reperfusion, underscoring the importance of timely cooling relative to the end of ischemia and onset of reperfusion. Dae et al. investigated the impact of cooling on myocardial infarction using a human-sized pig model. Here, systemic cooling via an endovascular temperature catheter commenced 20 minutes into a 60-minute coronary occlusion and continued with gradual rewarming during the subsequent 3-hour reperfusion period. Although the area at risk (AAR) was similar in both hypothermic ($19 \pm 3\%$) and normothermic ($20 \pm 7\%$) subjects, there was a significant reduction in infarct size among the hypothermic group ($9 \pm 6\%$ vs. $45 \pm 8\%$). This protective effect of hypothermia partly stems from mitigated reperfusion injury, attributed to decreased myocardial oxygen consumption and slower ATP depletion rates during ischemia. This may also involve reduced release of vasodilatory mediators and altered responsiveness in endothelial and vascular smooth muscle cells. Shao et al. proposed that a critical acceleration of myocardial death occurs within the first hour of reperfusion, initiated by an immediate surge of oxidants and cytochrome c release upon reperfusion.

Clinical Trials

Numerous clinical studies on humans have been carried out to assess the impact of hypothermia in decreasing infarct size and preventing heart failure (HF) in acute myocardial infarction patients. These studies predominantly applied mild hypothermia, setting the temperature between 32–34°C, alongside adjuvant percutaneous coronary intervention (PCI) therapy. The COOL-MI InCor Trial explored the use of cooling as a supplementary treatment during PCI for AMI, employing endovascular methods to achieve a target hypothermia of approximately $32 \pm 1°C$. However, when hypothermia was applied to patients with anterior MI at temperatures below 35°C, there was a notable reduction in infarct size (9.3% vs. control 18.2%).

A smaller pilot study, Rapid MI-ICE, which involved rapid cooling using 4°C cold saline infusion maintained at 33°C for three hours, demonstrated a 38% reduction in infarct size relative to AAR, without subsequent development of HF. Another larger scale study, the CHILL-MI Trial, aimed to quickly induce hypothermia at 33°C for one hour but failed to show an overall decrease in infarct size/AAR, although it did report a 33% reduction in infarct size on the anterior wall and a lower rate of HF after 45 days (3% vs. 14% in controls).

The VELOCITY trial, utilizing an automated peritoneal lavage device for inducing mild hypothermia below 35°C, yielded inconclusive outcomes with no significant changes in infarct size or microvascular obstruction, and an increase in major cardiac adverse events within the first 30 days. Notably, this method also extended the door-to-balloon time by approximately 15 minutes and led to stent thrombosis exclusively in the hypothermia group, suggesting that the risks associated with peritoneal cooling and prolonged ischemia might outweigh the benefits of preventing ischemia/reperfusion injury through hypothermia.

Conversely, the COOL AMI EU pilot trial, which also focused on cooling as an adjunct therapy during PCI in AMI patients, achieved a significant reduction in infarct size relative to left ventricular mass by up to 30% in anterior STEMI (ST-Elevation Myocardial Infarction) patients (16.7% vs. 23.8% in controls). This trial utilized a rapid cooling protocol that reached 33.6°C during reperfusion and reduced the temperature by over 1.1°C compared to earlier trials, with a reperfusion delay of only 17 minutes due to cooling. Furthermore, research by Villablanca et al. indicated that hypothermia primarily benefits those with anterior wall MI by reducing infarct size, but it does not significantly affect major adverse cardiac events (MACE) or mortality rates [39].

Possible Mechanism of TH After MI

The primary principle behind the cardioprotective effects of cooling is the conservation of energy; this includes 1) lowering the metabolic needs of the myocardium which helps in preserving adenosine triphosphate and glycogen, 2) improving cellular membrane stability due to decreased acidosis, 3) mitigating the overload of $Na+$ and Ca^{2+}, and 4) bolstering mitochondrial membrane stability through the inhibition of calcium-induced openings of the mitochondrial permeability transition pore (MPTP); this also helps in maintaining ion balance during ischemic and reperfusion phases, and in preserving microvascular structures. Observations have shown that cooling has positive impacts on mitochondria in both non-reperfused and reperfused myocardial tissues. Tissier and colleagues found that under non-reperfused conditions, the Ca^{2+} concentration needed to trigger MPTP opening was slightly lower in cooled hearts (-16%) compared to a -49% reduction in normothermic hearts. In ischemia-reperfusion conditions, significant reductions were noted in both cooled (-37%) and control (-68%) hearts, with a more pronounced decrease in the latter. The protective mechanism is suggested to involve enhancement of the ERK signaling pathway during ischemia, whereas protection associated with pre-/post conditioning relies on ERK activation in the initial moments of reperfusion [38].

Hypothermia Causes Energy Preservation

The cardioprotective mechanisms of therapeutic hypothermia have long been attributed to its ability to decrease metabolism and conserve energy. For instance, employing cold cardioplegia (below 20°C) leads to a significant drop in cardiac metabolic activity and helps maintain levels of adenosine triphosphate. Similarly, mild hypothermia (32—34°C) has been observed to lower ATP depletion in both isolated hearts under ischemic conditions and in regional ischemia in vivo, although the effect is less pronounced than with deeper hypothermia (below 31°C). Intriguingly, in vitro experiments indicate that the relationship between temperature reduction and energy conservation is not directly proportional; ATP and glucose utilization remain nearly unchanged when temperatures are sustained above 35°C. Nevertheless, maintaining a temperature of 35°C continues to effectively reduce infarct size, implying that therapeutic hypothermia may exert its beneficial effects through additional pathways beyond mere metabolic slowdown. This perspective is further supported by studies demonstrating that blocking the extracellular signal-regulated kinase survival pathway does not impact the ATP-conserving capacity of hypothermia, yet it eliminates its ability to reduce infarct size in isolated rabbit hearts. These findings suggest that metabolic adjustments might not fully account for the cardioprotective benefits of hypothermia. Moreover, it was previously theorized that hypothermia-induced bradycardia might contribute to energy conservation in vivo and enhance ischemic tolerance. However, this theory was refuted by evidence showing that cardiac pacing at elevated heart rates does not negate the cardioprotective effects of hypothermia.

The Effect of Hypothermia Implementation on Mitochondria and Reactive Oxygen Species

Mitochondria have long been recognized as a key focus for the cardioprotective effects of hypothermia, extending beyond the previously discussed metabolic adjustments. It is established that mitochondrial electron transport and respiratory functions are significantly affected by temperature changes. For example, the respiratory control ratio shows marked improvement in isolated rabbit cardiac mitochondria at 32°C compared to 38°C, with an increase of 22% under normoxic conditions. Simultaneously, there is a substantial reduction in the production of reactive oxygen species at 32°C versus 38°C, showing a decrease of 41% under similar conditions. In isolated rat cardiomyocytes, the production of reactive oxygen species notably drops during hypoxia at 32°C compared to 38°C, with a reduction of 55% after 140 minutes of hypoxia.

Furthermore, hypothermia helps alleviate dysfunctions in mitochondrial complexes I, II, and III in rabbits undergoing 30 minutes of coronary artery occlusion. This protective effect also limits the generation of mitochondrial reactive oxygen species and the associated oxidative stress, as evidenced by reduced lipid peroxidation. Hypothermia also influences the mitochondrial permeability transition pore (mPTP), a critical element in cardioprotective strategies. This was examined in rabbits subjected to 30 minutes of coronary artery occlusion, where myocardial mitochondria were analyzed just before reperfusion (ischemic mitochondria) and five minutes post-reperfusion (reperfused mitochondria). The studies indicated that hypothermia enhances the mitochondrial capacity to regulate calcium at the end of the ischemic period but does not counteract the heightened sensitivity triggered by reperfusion. Thus, while hypothermia effectively prevents mPTP opening during ischemia, it does not alleviate reperfusion injuries. This observation aligns with physiological findings that hypothermia does not significantly reduce infarct size upon reperfusion. This contrasts with ischemic preconditioning, which effectively blocks mPTP opening during reperfusion by activating reperfusion-induced salvaged kinase pathways.

The Effect of Hypothermia on Signaling Pathways

Numerous experimental investigations have sought to understand the mechanisms underlying hypothermia and their potential connection to specific signaling pathways. This research holds significant promise, particularly if the protective effects of hypothermia could be replicated through pharmacological means. These mechanistic insights have been comprehensively reviewed elsewhere. To summarize a decrease in temperature has been demonstrated to trigger the Akt pathways and activate heat-shock proteins 27 or 70 in mouse cardiomyocytes subjected to artificial ischemia. Similarly, the involvement of ERKs has been established in isolated rabbit hearts experiencing regional ischemia. Here, the protective effects of mild hypothermia (35°C) were completely negated by two distinct ERK inhibitors. Notably, ERK inhibition did not impact ATP levels, indicating that the preservation of energy might not be directly linked to the cardioprotective effects of hypothermia. Consequently, further research is essential to deepen our understanding of hypothermia's anti-ischemic properties and to identify new targets for replicating its cardioprotective benefits [40].

The Effect of Therapeutic Hypothermia on Microvascular Obstruction

Beyond reducing the size of infarcts, therapeutic hypothermia has also been found to positively influence post-reperfusion coronary flow. In their research, Hale and colleagues observed that applying ice bag cooling directly to the hearts of rabbits during the peri-reperfusion phase diminished the no-reflow phenomenon, while not altering the size of acute infarcts. Supporting these findings, Gotberg and associates conducted experiments on pigs, revealing a notable decrease in microvascular obstruction within ischemic regions, as determined by single photon emission computed tomography. Nevertheless, these promising results have not yet been consistently replicated in human clinical trials. One particular randomized study did not observe any significant differences in microvascular obstruction sizes between hypothermia-treated patients and control subjects. Similarly, recent work by Testori and colleagues using cardiac magnetic resonance imaging showed no significant differences in the areas of microvascular obstruction between groups treated with or without TH four days following the onset of STEMI.

TH for Cardiogenic Shock Associated with STEMI

As previously mentioned, mild therapeutic hypothermia enhances cardiac contractility. It also causes vasoconstriction in the peripheral blood vessels, which elevates systemic vascular resistance and subsequently increases arterial pressure. Additionally, systemic hypothermia lowers the metabolic requirements of the entire body, thereby balancing the oxygen supply and demand for non-cardiac organs. Consequently, hypothermia could theoretically serve as an effective treatment for cardiogenic shock. Clinical observations following cardiac surgeries have shown that hypothermia elevates venous oxygen saturation, suggesting an optimization of oxygen utilization across the body. However, a post-hoc analysis of the TTM trial indicated a higher prevalence of patients requiring substantial vasopressor support in the 33°C group compared to the 36°C group. The implications of this for cardiogenic shock patients are yet to be determined. In a recent randomized study of 40 cardiogenic shock patients, hypothermia did not enhance cardiac power or overall clinical outcomes. Since only about half of these patients had STEMI-related cardiogenic shock, further research is necessary to assess the safety and effectiveness of hypothermia in treating this specific subgroup.

Potential Reasons for Lack of Efficacy in Clinical Trials

While it is anticipated that blood temperature would align with the temperature of the heart during cardiac events, directly measuring the temperature of ischemic myocardial tissue in the context of STEMI proves to be a complex task. Additionally, the rate at which the heart and other organs are cooled can vary significantly based on the method used. Consequently, the ambiguous outcomes observed in previous studies may stem from inadequate reduction of temperature in ischemic myocardial regions compared to the temperatures that were recorded. In contrast to animal studies where direct measurement of infarct size is possible, human studies typically rely on imaging techniques to estimate infarct size, which could introduce errors into these measurements and potentially confound the findings. Furthermore, some patients experiencing STEMI may have already undergone reperfusion by the time their initial coronary angiogram is conducted. According to recent findings by Dae et al. and supporting preclinical research, these patients might not derive benefit from therapeutic hypothermia if reperfusion has occurred prior to intervention. It is also important to consider that the effectiveness of certain medications can be diminished at lower body temperatures, necessitating careful management of drug interactions. Additionally, there is potential for TH to enhance the effects of other treatments aimed at minimizing myocardial infarction damage, though this possibility remains largely uninvestigated [41].

Future Directions

Regarding the efficacy of reducing the size of an infarct, achieving a lower body temperature yields better outcomes. Mild therapeutic hypothermia, typically maintained between 32 to 35°C, is well tolerated in both mammals and humans. Therefore, reaching a target temperature as low as 32°C is crucial for maximizing the reduction of infarct size in patients with acute myocardial infarction. Key areas for improvement include: 1) Development of clinically suitable devices and pharmaceuticals, 2) Enhancement of protocols and medical support throughout the cooling and rewarming phases, and 3) Expansion of cooling technology options and addressing safety concerns, such as the use of localized cooling devices, to reliably achieve the target temperature of 32°C [38].

Conclusion

Numerous randomized controlled trials and combined analyses have utilized both intravenous cold saline infusion and endovascular cooling catheters. These studies confirm the feasibility of therapeutic hypothermia for protecting the heart during acute myocardial infarction. Echoing findings from experimental research, these RCTs demonstrate that rapid and early application of TH at the onset of reperfusion significantly reduces infarct size. Moreover, even a slight delay in applying TH can still effectively reduce the frequency of post-infarction heart failure. TH is particularly beneficial in cases involving large areas of myocardium at risk and anterior wall infarctions. Therefore, it is crucial to initiate cooling promptly without postponing reperfusion treatment to ensure optimal outcomes. The diversification of cooling technologies and the use of experienced medical teams could enhance the rate of cooling without increasing the risk of complications, while also achieving the target temperature of 32°C. Initial cooling methods might include topical surface cooling or transnasal evaporative cooling, which can be used alongside more rapid cooling techniques such as endovascular catheters. Further experimental research is necessary to develop optimal strategies that include clinically viable devices and pharmaceuticals. Additionally, larger and more comprehensive RCTs involving AMI patients are essential to advance this field.

Chapter 11

Hypothermia Implementation in Acute Liver Failure

Acute liver failure (ALF) is characterized by severe hepatocellular injury occurring without any prior liver disease, making it a devastating and often fatal condition. While the injury may be reversible, clinical progression frequently leads to multiple organ failure, which carries a poor prognosis. The incidence of ALF ranges from 1 to 6 cases per million people annually. However, this information primarily reflects data from developed countries [42].

How Should Subjects Be Cooled?

In individuals suffering from ALF and ICH, current research supports the prompt application of hypothermia for optimal impact on ICP management. In populations without ALF, endovascular cooling methods typically reach target temperatures faster than external methods like cooling blankets or jackets, and they offer the advantage of simultaneously monitoring core temperature through the same catheter. However, ALF patients present differently compared to those with traumatic brain injury or cardiac arrest due to significant cutaneous vasodilation, which facilitates highly effective heat dissipation using external cooling methods. Initial studies involving ALF patients have demonstrated that target temperatures can be reached within one hour using cooling blankets. Additional factors, including a tendency towards bleeding and a higher susceptibility to infections in ALF patients, further indicate that external cooling devices might be a preferable choice for administering hypothermia safely [43].

To What Temperature Should Patients Be Cooled

Initial investigations into the use of hypothermia for acute liver failure patients have generally maintained core temperatures between 32–33°C, aligning with protocols used in other medical conditions. However, it is critical to avoid reducing core temperatures below 30°C due to the significant risk of infections and cardiac dysrhythmias. Excessive cooling can also potentially hinder liver regeneration, a factor that needs to be weighed against the benefits of reducing intracranial pressure and enhancing neurological outcomes in ALF patients. Unfortunately, there is a lack of dose-response data in this patient group to guide optimal cooling levels.

Duration of Hypothermia in ALF Patients

In earlier studies, ALF patients have tolerated up to approximately five days of hypothermia without negative outcomes. Nonetheless, extended periods of reduced body temperature increase the likelihood of complications, especially infections. Prolonged hypothermia should therefore be reserved for specific situations such as pending orthotopic liver transplantation (OLT), and is less advisable for non-OLT candidates. It is observed that liver regeneration from ALF due to acetaminophen (APAP) overdose typically occurs within 72 hours, faster than other causes of ALF. Consequently, a cooling period of 72 hours may be an appropriate target to evaluate the therapeutic impact on ICP for non-OLT candidates, whereas longer durations might be justified for those awaiting transplantation.

Re-Warming Strategy for Hypothermic ALF Patients

Re-warming ALF patients' post-hypothermia treatment introduces several hazards. These include exacerbating electrolyte imbalances—a common complication in ALF—and inducing vasodilation which can further reduce mean arterial pressure. This poses a heightened risk of decreasing cerebral perfusion pressure (CPP) and potentially leading to cerebral ischemia. Literature on safe re-warming rates varies from 1°C per hour to 1°C per day in the context of traumatic brain injuries. Although specific re-warming rates for ALF patients are not well-documented, a cautious approach would be a gradual increase in temperature, potentially at a rate of 1°C every 12 hours.

Improvements in treating patients with acute liver failure have resulted in lower rates of occurrence and mortality related to cerebral edema and intracranial hypertension. Additionally, these conditions are responsible for significant mortality rates (ranging from 25% to 50%) and can lead to neurocognitive impairments in those who survive. Increasing experimental and clinical evidence supports the use of mild hypothermia (maintaining body temperature between 32 and 35 degrees Celsius) as a crucial intervention to prevent cerebral edema and intracranial hypertension in cases of fulminant hepatic failure. This cooling technique has been found to mitigate or even reverse many of the pathophysiological processes that contribute to cerebral edema in ALF.

The protective effects of hypothermia on liver damage were initially recognized in 1962, demonstrating its effectiveness against acute ammonia toxicity in mice. Subsequently, Traber et al. observed that natural occurrences of hypothermia in a rat model of ALF led to significant reductions in both cerebral edema and the onset of encephalopathy, compared to rats kept at a normal body temperature. This protective phenomenon has since been confirmed in various other animal models of ALF, suggesting that hypothermia's ability to positively influence multiple injury pathways is key to its consistent and notable success in reducing cerebrovascular complications in experimental ALF. The primary mechanisms by which hypothermia is thought to be effective include lowering systemic and brain ammonia levels and reducing cerebral blood flow. However, numerous other systemic and cerebrovascular benefits have also been suggested to contribute to its efficacy.

Hypothermia, without alterations in circulating ammonia levels, independently reduces ammonia concentrations in both the brain and cerebrospinal fluid of mice. Additionally, elevated ammonia levels in the brain disrupt normal glucose metabolism, leading to increased production of glutamine and heightened oxidative stress. Disruptions in glucose metabolism result in enhanced activity along the glycolytic pathway and a rise in lactate synthesis. In animal studies of acute liver failure, hypothermia was shown to reduce the production of lactate and alanine, subsequently diminishing cerebral edema before these reductions occurred. These findings indicate that hypothermia can correct glucose metabolism disturbances in the brain. Although glutamine is often identified as a critical factor in ammonia metabolism linked to osmotic imbalances and fluid accumulation in the brain, hypothermia's prevention of brain edema did not coincide with lowered glutamine levels in ALF models. Nevertheless, hypothermia did significantly ameliorate disruptions in other osmolytes such as myo-inositol, taurine, glutamate, lactate, and alanine, thus enhancing the osmotic balance within the brain. Furthermore, hypothermia in animal models has been observed to reduce extracellular brain levels of glutamate and other amino acids, as glutamate typically rises in both human patients and experimental models of ALF. Hypothermia also exhibits notable anti-inflammatory effects; inflammatory mediators can exacerbate ammonia's toxicity, aggravating cerebral edema. Elevated levels of protein and mRNA markers for pro-inflammatory cytokines like IL-1 beta, TNF alpha, and IL-6 have been detected in the brains of rats undergoing hepatic devascularization during cerebral edema episodes. Hypothermia has been linked to decreased efflux of these cytokines in the brain of patients and reduced cytokine production and brain edema in animal studies. Moreover, lower body temperatures have been associated with decreased indicators of oxidative and nitrosative stress in the brain in animal models of ALF.

Negative impacts of acute liver failure on cerebrovascular hemodynamics are manifested by an increase in cerebral blood flow and a disruption of cerebrovascular autoregulation. This is due to both absolute and relative increases in cerebral blood flow compared to cerebral metabolic needs, contributing to the onset of cerebral edema and elevated intracranial pressure. Therapeutic hypothermia can counter these effects by reducing cerebral blood flow and reinstating autoregulation in ALF patients. Additionally, in cases where cerebral edema and heightened ICP are resistant to standard medical treatments, hypothermia not only reduces ICP but also re-establishes cerebrovascular autoregulation in response to changes in mean arterial pressure and enhances the vasodilatory response to alterations in carbon dioxide partial pressure.

Hypothermia has been shown to consistently decrease ammonia levels in both human subjects and animal models of ALF. Furthermore, in a specific experimental setup where hepatic detoxification was circumvented, hypothermia still managed to reduce systemic ammonia levels, indicating that ammonia production is temperature-dependent and potentially more sensitive to temperature changes than detoxification processes. ALF typically presents with distributive physiology, characterized by increased cardiac output and reduced systemic vascular resistance. The activation of the systemic inflammatory response syndrome is crucial in the hemodynamic disturbances observed in ALF. Inflammation, in conjunction with ammonia, contributes to the elevation of ICP in individuals with ALF, likely through influencing cerebral blood flow. Hypothermia has been found to lower systemic pro-inflammatory cytokines in both animal studies and ALF patients. Moreover, hypothermia positively affects systemic hemodynamics. Clinical studies in ALF patients with high ICP have shown that inducing hypothermia raises systemic vascular resistance and reduces the cardiac output, thereby reducing the need for vasopressors [44]. The onset of brain edema and elevated intracranial pressure (ICP) are distinctive complications observed in patients with acute liver failure who experience severe hepatic encephalopathy.

Brain Ammonia

In acute liver failure, the ratio of ammonia in the blood to that in the brain can increase by up to eight times the normal level. This rise in brain ammonia is crucial for the onset of brain edema in ALF as it disrupts normal brain glucose metabolism, enhances glutamine production in astrocytes, and induces oxidative/nitrosative stress among other changes. Studies have demonstrated that lowering body temperature can reduce ammonia levels in both the brain and cerebrospinal fluid. This effect was observed in mice administered with ammonium chloride and in rats undergoing hepatic devascularization, without alterations in ammonia levels in the bloodstream. The decrease in cerebral blood flow (CBF) caused by hypothermia may significantly contribute to these effects, although a direct influence of hypothermia on how ammonia is metabolized in the brain might also play a role.

Brain Glucose Metabolism

Changes in brain glucose metabolism, typical of acute liver failure and hyperammonemia, are believed to play a crucial role in the onset of brain edema and elevated intracranial pressure. Additionally, there has been evidence of increased glycolytic activity in glucose processing leading to heightened lactate production in rat models with hepatic artery ligation. Similarly, elevated lactate levels have been noted in the extracellular fluid of the brain in ALF patients, often occurring before spikes in ICP. It is also significant that a reduction in brain energy metabolism, marked by decreased cerebral metabolic rates of glucose and oxygen, constitutes a primary consequence of hypothermia. In cases of ALF where therapeutic hypothermia is applied, the decline in cerebral metabolic rate for glucose exceeds that of oxygen, indicating a potential enhancement in brain oxidative metabolism (Jalan et al. 1999b). In experimental settings involving rats with hepatic devascularization, lowering body temperature by 2°C effectively halted the increased synthesis of lactate and alanine and reduced lactate levels in the cerebrospinal fluid. These changes occurred before hypothermia's mitigating effects on brain edema were observed. These findings underscore the efficacy of hypothermia in moderating significant disruptions in brain glucose metabolism seen in ALF.

Disruption of Brain Osmotic Balance

In the brain, the enzyme glutamine synthetase metabolizes ammonia rapidly within astrocytes, leading to an intracellular build-up of glutamine. This accumulation is believed to induce osmotic swelling, known as the glutamine hypothesis, and triggers a compensatory reduction in other organic osmolytes. The issue of glutamine build-up in acute liver failure is multifaceted, with newer studies indicating that glutamine may also accumulate in astrocytes due to reduced activity of the high-affinity glutamine transporter SNAT5. Additionally, other substances like alanine and lactate, which increase in the brain during ALF, might further exacerbate osmotic disturbances in the brain. Intriguingly, while mild hypothermia has been shown to prevent brain edema, it does not appear to reduce glutamine accumulation in the brain, as observed in experiments involving portacaval-shunted rats treated with ammonia and rats with ALF caused by hepatic devascularization. However, these studies also noted that mild hypothermia significantly mitigated changes in other brain osmolytes, including the depletion of myo-inositol, taurine, and glutamate, and the rise in alanine and lactate levels, pointing towards an overall improvement in brain osmotic balance.

Concentration of Amino Acids in the Brain's Extracellular Space

ALF leads to significant changes in the brain's glutamate system, notably a marked reduction in its overall levels. In contrast, the amount of glutamate in the extracellular space of the brain tends to rise, as observed in both human patients and animal studies on ALF. This increase is likely due to enhanced release coupled with reduced uptake by astrocytes. The application of hypothermia has been shown to curb the ongoing rise of extracellular brain glutamate seen in normothermic rats undergoing hepatic devascularization. Furthermore, hypothermia helps reduce swelling in glutamate-stimulated astrocytes in laboratory settings. In cases of hepatic devascularization in rats, mild hypothermia further mitigates additional shifts in the makeup of the brain's extracellular fluid, including elevated levels of glycine and aromatic amino acids. This suggests that maintaining the normal balance of brain extracellular fluid could be another pathway through which hypothermia lessens the neurological impacts of ALF.

Brain Microglial Activation

Assessments of cerebral blood flow and arterio-venous differentials in the brain have revealed a significant release of pro-inflammatory cytokines in individuals with acute liver failure who experience elevated intracranial pressure. Concurrently, there has been a documented increase in both mRNA and protein levels of IL-1b, TNF-a, IL-6, along with signs of microglial activation in the brains of rats subjected to hepatic devascularization coinciding with brain edema. Furthermore, initiating mild hypothermia has been linked to decreased efflux of these pro-inflammatory cytokines in ALF patients, as well as reduced microglial activity, diminished cytokine production in the brain, and alleviation of brain edema in rat models of hepatic devascularization. These findings suggest that the anti-inflammatory effects of mild hypothermia could play a role in its therapeutic benefits for ALF.

Other Factors in the Brain

Additional brain changes in acute liver failure that could potentially be mitigated by hypothermia include the onset of oxidative/nitrosative stress, seizure episodes, and variations in gene expression. Notably, the accumulation of oxidative/nitrosative stress within astrocytes appears to be a critical phase in ammonia toxicity, which might be exacerbated by inflammatory mediators. Similar to findings in experimental stroke and inflammation studies, lowering body temperature has been shown to reduce indirect indicators of oxidative/nitrosative stress in rat models with hepatic devascularization. This includes decreases in nitrite/nitrate levels and mRNA levels of hemeoxygenase-1, inducible nitric oxide synthase (NOS), and endothelial NOS. However, in ALF patients, although therapeutic hypothermia lowered arterial levels of nitrite/nitrate and malondialdehyde, the cerebral outflow of these substances was nearly unchanged, making it difficult to confirm a reduction in brain oxidative/nitrosative stress. Subclinical seizures have also been suggested as a factor increasing the likelihood of brain edema in ALF. Although no direct studies have been conducted on ALF in this context, the application of hypothermia has effectively halted seizure activities in cases of refractory status epilepticus and diminished neuronal synchronization in stimulated hippocampal slices from rats, indicating another potential beneficial mechanism of hypothermia in ALF. Furthermore, inducing mild hypothermia in rats with hepatic devascularization restored normal brain gene expression for several proteins that were disrupted under normothermic conditions. These proteins include glial fibrillary acidic protein, the peripheral-type benzodiazepine receptor, hemeoxygenase-1, among others. Identifying which gene expression changes are mechanistically significant remains an area for further investigation.

Systemic Hemodynamics

Individuals suffering from acute liver failure typically exhibit a hyperdynamic circulatory state, marked by elevated cardiac output, rapid heart rate, and reduced systemic vascular resistance. This condition can escalate to hemodynamic instability and shock, contributing significantly to the onset of renal failure and other ALF-related complications. A pivotal study by Jalan et al. highlighted that implementing therapeutic hypothermia in ALF patients with elevated intracranial pressure led to normalization of cardiac output and heart rate, along with increased systemic vascular resistance. Interestingly, this intervention did not alter mean arterial pressure, yet it substantially decreased the need for noradrenaline to maintain safe arterial pressure levels during mild hypothermia. Furthermore, maintaining therapeutic hypothermia during emergency liver transplantation has been shown to improve hemodynamic control throughout the surgical process. These findings suggest that the hemodynamic benefits of therapeutic hypothermia may provide substantial advantages in managing ALF, potentially easing the management of hemodynamics and mitigating additional peripheral complications.

Systemic Inflammation

Patients with acute liver failure from any cause typically exhibit systemic inflammation, which is directly linked to the increased risk of morbidity and mortality associated with the condition. This inflammation not only exacerbates liver damage but also leads to hemodynamic instability and numerous other complications in ALF. The anti-inflammatory effects of hypothermia have been well-documented across various medical scenarios beyond ALF. In cases of ALF accompanied by elevated intracranial pressure, the application of therapeutic hypothermia has been shown to significantly reduce levels of pro-inflammatory cytokines such as IL-1b, TNF-a, and IL-6. These findings are supported by experimental ALF models, including rats subjected to hepatic devascularization and mice with azoxymethane-induced liver damage. Notably, the production of certain cytokines like the anti-inflammatory IL-10 remains unchanged by hypothermia, suggesting a selective regulatory role of hypothermia on systemic inflammation. These collective findings underscore the potential therapeutic benefits of hypothermia in managing systemic inflammation in ALF [45].

Chapter 12

Therapeutic Hypothermia in Ischemic Stroke

Therapeutic Hypothermia in Experimental Ischemic Stroke

Recent experimental research has established that therapeutic hypothermia provides neuroprotection by positively influencing a wide array of pathological pathways. These include the regulation of apoptosis, brain metabolism, activation of microglia, cerebral blood flow, inflammation, and neurotrophic factors. Consequently, reducing brain temperature is believed to be crucial for the preservation of brain tissue and functionality.

The Effect of Hypothermia on Brain Metabolism

In models of ischemic stroke, applying mild hypothermia at around 33°C has been shown to enhance cerebral blood flow and maintain cellular metabolic rates. During a stroke, cerebral blood flow is initially interrupted due to vessel blockage. Upon reperfusion, or the restoration of blood flow, there is an initial excessive increase in blood flow which gradually worsens. This worsening has been attributed to microvascular constriction. Therapeutic hypothermia has been effective not only in enhancing and stabilizing cerebral blood flow by averting microcirculatory failure but also in preventing the initial excessive surge in blood flow following reperfusion.

Furthermore, brain metabolism exhibits sensitivity to changes in temperature. Mild hypothermia has been observed to decrease oxygen consumption by about 5% for each degree Celsius reduction in body temperature within the range of 22–37°C. Ischemic conditions in the brain also result in the heightened buildup of extracellular glutamate and an influx of calcium. Hypothermia has been proven to inhibit this accumulation of glutamate and the associated excitotoxic damage caused by calcium entry. More recent findings suggest that hypothermia may also diminish the expression of the calcium-sensing receptor (CaSR), which plays a role in regulating calcium entry, and enhances the expression of the inhibitory gamma-aminobutyric acid B receptor 1 (GABA-B-R1). Therefore, hypothermia is increasingly recognized for its capacity to exert neuroprotective effects in ischemia through its multifaceted impact on brain metabolism and neurotransmission.

Hypothermia as a Neuroprotective Strategy: Influencing Cell Death Mechanisms

Research has demonstrated that hypothermia can beneficially modify various pathways of ischemic cell death, including apoptosis. Numerous studies have confirmed that hypothermia helps prevent apoptotic cell death in experimental stroke models. Initially, therapeutic hypothermia was found to impact multiple facets of the intrinsic apoptotic pathway, contributing to neuroprotection. This pathway begins in the cell's mitochondria, which emit several factors like cytochrome c and apoptosis-inducing factor into the cytosol. Additionally, mild hypothermia has been observed to elevate levels of the anti-apoptotic protein Bcl-2. This increase in Bcl-2 subsequently blocks the release of cytochrome c into the cytosol and prevents the activation of caspases. Studies also suggest that mild hypothermia diminishes the production of the pro-apoptotic protein Bax. Beyond Bcl-2, hypothermia affects members of the protein kinase C (PKC) family, which includes types that promote and inhibit apoptosis, thereby decreasing apoptotic cell death.

The extrinsic apoptotic pathway, which is activated through death receptors, also plays a role in cell fate. A key receptor in this pathway, Fas, along with its ligand FasL, has been explored in stroke research, revealing that disruption of this pathway enhances outcomes. Hypothermia has been shown to lower the expression of both Fas and FasL, leading to reduced activation of caspase-8 involved in this pathway. Moreover, TH influences caspase-independent apoptotic processes. Specifically, it has been shown to inhibit the movement of AIF from the mitochondria to the cytosol, thus decreasing apoptosis in models of ischemic stroke. In conclusion, TH has a significant impact on various cell death mechanisms, promoting cellular survival across different pathways.

Hypothermia and Cell Survival Pathways

Therapeutic hypothermia and its effects on cellular mechanisms present a fascinating dichotomy. While TH is known to suppress various molecules that promote apoptotic cell death, it simultaneously enhances the expression of multiple cell survival factors. This dual effect may be partially attributed to the activation of cold stress proteins, which are produced in response to reduced body temperatures. Among these proteins, RNA-binding motif protein 3 (RBM3) is particularly noteworthy. Extensively researched, RBM3 levels have been observed to rise during hypothermic conditions following a stroke, as evidenced by both laboratory and clinical research, and is linked to neuroprotective outcomes.

Furthermore, TH has been demonstrated to boost levels of several neurotrophic factors such as brain-derived neurotrophic factor (BDNF), glial-derived neurotrophic factor (GDNF), and neurotrophin (NT) in brain tissues damaged by ischemia. Additionally, mild hypothermia is known to trigger the phosphorylation of extracellular signal-regulated kinase-1/2 (ERK1/2), a process that occurs downstream of BDNF signaling. TH also activates Akt, a serine/threonine protein kinase that plays crucial roles in cell plasticity and migration. In the signaling cascade downstream of Akt, the phosphatase and tensin homolog (PTEN) typically leads to apoptosis. However, when phosphorylated, PTEN supports cell survival instead. This phosphorylated form of PTEN is critical in preventing neuronal cell death in ischemic brain injuries. In models of stroke, TH has been shown to maintain elevated levels of phosphorylated PTEN, suggesting that while cooling the brain may reduce metabolic and cellular activities, it also facilitates the enhancement of mechanisms that foster cell survival.

Anti-Inflammatory Impacts of Therapeutic Hypothermia

After an acute ischemic stroke, necrotic cells, cellular debris, and a surge in reactive oxygen species (ROS) trigger inflammatory reactions. These reactions involve the activation of microglia and the migration of leukocytes from the bloodstream into the brain's parenchymal tissue. This movement of immune cells from both the brain and periphery to the site of ischemia can intensify and broaden the scope of the infarct [61]. Mild hypothermia has been found to inhibit microglial activation and enhance tissue viability following ischemic stroke [35], as well as block neutrophils from penetrating ischemic brain regions. Therapeutic hypothermia is also effective in lowering various inflammatory mediators, including adhesion molecules, ROS, and pro-inflammatory cytokines [62–64].

Furthermore, TH influences the activity of key transcription factors that drive inflammatory responses, such as nuclear factor-kB (NF-kB) [65]. In models of brain ischemia, TH has prevented the migration of NF-kB into the nucleus and inhibited the activation of related pro-inflammatory genes [66]. Additionally, TH has been shown to suppress other transcription factors like mitogen-activated protein kinase (MAPK) and Janus kinases/signal transducer and activator of transcription proteins (JAK/STATs), which are known to promote inflammation after a stroke [67, 68].

Cytokines, crucial for immune system communication and enhancing immune responses, are rapidly and significantly upregulated in brain tissue post-stroke [69]. TH has been effective in reducing many inflammatory cytokines, such as transforming growth factor (TGF)-b, tumor necrosis factor (TNF-a), and various interleukins [59, 64]. It has also induced an anti-inflammatory M2 phenotype in microglia within stroke models [70]. Recent studies have indicated that maintaining a normal body temperature around 36°C can lower the levels of several pro-inflammatory cytokines [71], and adjusting temperature to either 33°C or 36°C has been equally beneficial in neuroprotection. This is achieved by diminishing pro-inflammatory M1 microglial activation and promoting a shift towards a protective M2 microglial phenotype [71]. Given recent clinical concerns that therapeutic hypothermia to temperatures between 32–34°C may not be well tolerated by some patients, maintaining a body temperature at 36°C could be more acceptable clinically and still offer therapeutic and anti-inflammatory benefits.

Optimal Target Temperature

Hypothermia was found to decrease infarct size by more than 40% when temperatures were maintained at 34°C or lower. Even a modest reduction to 35°C still led to a significant reduction in infarct size, approximately 30% (with a 95% confidence interval ranging from 21% to 39%), indicating that even slight cooling could serve as an effective neuroprotective measure. Subsequent research not covered in this review assessed the effects of cooling at temperatures of 36°C, 35°C, 34°C, 33°C, and 32°C for four hours, initiated 90 minutes following occlusion of the middle cerebral artery in rats, compared to a normothermic control of 37°C. Results showed that only reductions to 34°C and 33°C improved outcomes, with the greatest benefits seen at 34°C, pointing to this temperature as the ideal target for therapeutic hypothermia in treating acute ischemic stroke. Additionally, lowering body temperature to 35.5°C or 35°C has proven both practical and safe for conscious patients suffering from acute ischemic stroke through external cooling methods, used alongside pethidine to manage shivering.

Duration of Cooling

In studies involving animal models of localized brain ischemia, various pathophysiological mechanisms are triggered, each manifesting their harmful impacts over a span ranging from the initial hours to several days following the blockage of a blood vessel. A meta-analysis revealed a subtle yet surprising inverse correlation between the length of hypothermia application and its effectiveness. However, out of 277 experiments, 193 (70%) applied hypothermia for just a few hours, and only 32 (12%) extended this cooling period beyond 12 hours, making it difficult to draw definitive conclusions about the advantages of prolonged hypothermia. Moreover, two separate studies that compared longer cooling periods (over 12 hours) with shorter ones (less than 12 hours) reported significantly better outcomes with extended cooling durations.

In another experiment, cooling rats to 33°C starting one hour after permanent occlusion of the middle cerebral artery showed that maintaining hypothermia for 48 hours resulted in superior functional and structural outcomes compared to shorter durations of 24 or 12 hours, with the least benefit observed in the shortest cooling period. According to pre-clinical research, timing is crucial in treating cerebral ischemia. A combined analysis of six randomized trials using intravenous thrombolysis with rt-PA strongly indicated that earlier treatment initiation within 6 hours post-stroke led to better outcomes. Limited clinical data exist on the use of therapeutic cooling in cases of intracerebral hemorrhage (ICH), but findings from a small nonrandomized study suggest that mild hypothermia (35°C), initiated more than 12 hours after the onset of ICH and maintained for 10 days, may decrease mortality rates without increasing the risk of further bleeding.

Brain Cooling

Utilizing whole body cooling to reduce brain temperatures may unintentionally cause systemic issues. However, selective brain cooling offers a promising alternative that could circumvent these risks while providing substantial neuroprotection. This technique specifically cools the brain to a temperature below that of the body's core by creating a temperature differential between the two areas. Research has demonstrated its practicality and the similar benefits it shares with therapeutic hypothermia across various animal studies. For stroke patients, in particular, selective brain cooling presents a viable option for neuroprotection compared to full-body hypothermia. Selective brain cooling achieves quicker, more targeted cooling and stabilization of the brain's temperature than systemic hypothermia. Given the limited time available for intervention following ischemic events—ranging from minutes to hours—this method includes both non-invasive and invasive techniques. Non-invasive methods encompass localized surface cooling using devices like helmets, caps, or head-and-neck cooling units, which can establish an average temperature gradient of 3.4°C between the brain and the body core. Experiments on newborn pigs have validated the feasibility of selective brain cooling under conditions of global ischemic insult.

However, it is important to note that non-invasive methods such as surface and nasopharyngeal cooling are generally less effective at reducing the temperature of the brain tissue itself. Moreover, the process of surface cooling can induce a decrease in the temperature of circulating blood, which may facilitate the cooling of other body regions as well. Invasive techniques for selective cooling include methods such as subarachnoid, epidural and subdural cooling; intra-arterial selective cooling and retrograde jugular venous cooling. Although these invasive approaches are effective, they are associated with higher risks of infection and intracranial bleeding, which restrict their use in clinical environments.

In a small scale, non-randomized, observational studies, Chen et al. have shown that it is feasible and safe to reduce brain temperature by at least 2°C using an intra-arterial infusion of 4°C saline along with endovascular recanalization in patients experiencing acute ischemic stroke [46]. Additionally, a prospective non-randomized cohort study involving 113 patients with acute ischemic stroke indicated a reduction in infarct volume within 3–7 days post-treatment, maintaining acceptable safety levels in patients who underwent mechanical thrombectomy with an added intra-arterial selective cooling infusion. Nevertheless, no significant differences were observed at the 90-day mark in the percentage of patients achieving functional independence (mRS 0–2). The clinical efficacy of selective endovascular brain cooling in patients with large-vessel occlusions in ischemic stroke still requires further investigation. However, the integration of thrombolytic and mechanical recanalization therapies has been proven to enhance functional outcomes following acute stroke, suggesting that incorporating selective endovascular cooling could be seamlessly achieved in clinical practice. Combining selective brain cooling with recanalization might offer enhanced benefits, as preclinical studies suggest that therapeutic hypothermia is more effective when followed by reperfusion.

Recently, innovative selective cooling systems that merge nasopharyngeal brain and endovascular cooling technologies have been introduced. Advances in technology, including the use of smart devices, sensors and artificial intelligence hold promise for reducing complications and enhancing the effectiveness of selective brain cooling treatments. Further research is essential to develop optimal protocols for selective brain cooling that enhance clinical outcomes for stroke patients [47].

Chapter 13

The Implementation of Hypothermia in Traumatic Brain Injury

Traumatic brain injury (TBI) poses a significant public health challenge, affecting over 50 million individuals globally each year. TBI can lead to ischemic stroke, brain swelling (edema), increased intracranial pressure (ICP), and exacerbation of the injury. Cellular death may occur within minutes to hours following the trauma, with adverse effects potentially persisting for 72 hours or more. Therapeutic hypothermia has been shown to decrease ICP and act as a neuroprotective agent to some degree, thus preserving neuronal function, enhancing patient outcomes, and contributing to lower mortality rates. Despite this, the application of TH in TBI cases is still a subject of debate. Extensive animal research supports the use of TH, and various studies indicate that it can enhance neurological outcomes and decrease death rates. Nevertheless, recent research suggests that TH does not necessarily improve outcomes for patients with severe TBI compared to standard treatment. Furthermore, findings from a significant multicenter study indicate that TH may negatively impact both mortality rates and functional outcomes. Consequently, the use of TH in TBI management continues to be contentious [48].

Clinical Trials

In a study published in 1997 by Marion et al. 84 patients with severe traumatic brain injury (TBI) underwent treatment with mild hypothermia, maintained at 33°C for 24 hours. The findings indicated notably improved neurological outcomes at both three- and six-months post-treatment for those patients who had Glasgow Coma Scale (GCS) scores between 5 and 7 upon hospital admission. At the time of the review, no other treatment had shown such a pronounced neuroprotective effect for TBI patients. Later studies, including those by Clifton et al. involved larger patient groups (392 and 232 participants in 2001 and 2011, respectively, in the NABIS: H I & II trials) and tested early hypothermia initiation (within 2-5 hours). These studies concluded that therapeutic hypothermia did not alter neurological outcomes.

Further research by Jiang et al. in 2006 explored the timing of hypothermia application in TBI treatment. Their randomized trial with 215 severe TBI patients demonstrated that extended hypothermia duration (5 ± 1.3 days) led to fewer poor neurological outcomes compared to a shorter duration (2 ± 0.6 days). In both groups, cooling methods aimed to achieve rectal temperatures of 33–35°C using cooling blankets. A Cochrane review in 2009 by Kramer et al. which included 23 trials and 1,614 patients, assessed early hypothermia with target temperatures of at least 35°C for a minimum of 12 hours. The review suggested that hypothermia treatment was associated with better mortality rates and neurological outcomes, although this finding was significant only in studies deemed to be of lower methodological quality. The potential of hypothermia therapy in managing ongoing brain edema and refractory intracranial hypertension (IH) during the sub-acute phase of TBI has also been examined extensively. In 2003, Tokutomi et al. reported on 31 high-risk TBI patients with GCS scores of ≤5 at admission; nearly three-quarters required surgical intervention. Their findings supported the effectiveness of hypothermia in treating IH and highlighted optimal coupling between cerebral blood flow and metabolism at a temperature of 35°C without compromising perfusion pressure. Subsequent research by the same group compared outcomes at 35°C with those previously achieved at 33°C, revealing better control of brain perfusion pressure at the higher temperature without affecting ICP levels, complications, mortality, or neurological outcomes. The European Society of Intensive Care Medicine initiated a multicenter randomized clinical trial aiming to enroll 1,800 TBI patients to assess the benefits of therapeutic hypothermia (32–35°C) on ICP control, morbidity, and six-month mortality. The study did not specify a uniform duration for hypothermia application but suggested extending the cooling period as needed to maintain an ICP below 20 mmHg. A systematic review in 2012 encompassing 13 randomized clinical trials and five observational studies focused on IH management in TBI patients through therapeutic hypothermia. This review confirmed a significant reduction in ICP across all studied patients [49].

During the 1960s, profound hypothermia was frequently employed in hospitals to manage severe traumatic brain injury, but it was discontinued in the 1970s due to adverse effects such as infections, thrombosis, and arrhythmias that led to unsatisfactory treatment outcomes. Interest in hypothermic treatment for TBI resurfaced in the 1990s when various clinical trials indicated that a moderate level of hypothermia could enhance recovery in clinically relevant TBI models. This renewed interest was also linked to the prevention of cerebral hypoxia post-TBI, which is crucial for improving patient outcomes.

Successful applications of therapeutic hypothermia were reported where reductions in hypoxic incidents post-TBI were managed through strategies like brain tissue oxygen-guided cerebral perfusion pressure management combined with mild therapeutic hypothermia. In a study by Marion et al. they compared outcomes between hypothermic and normothermic treatments in 82 TBI patients. The findings showed that 62% of patients receiving hypothermia exhibited favorable outcomes, as opposed to 38% in the normothermic group.

Further research by Jiang et al. explored the impact of prolonged mild therapeutic hypothermia (lasting 3-14 days at temperatures between 33-35°C) on 87 patients with severe TBI. Their study revealed no significant difference in complication rates between the normothermic and hypothermic groups, though the latter displayed significantly reduced intracranial pressure (ICP) and lower levels of hyperglycemia. The duration of therapeutic hypothermia proved critical, with findings suggesting that cooling for five days resulted in better behavioral outcomes compared to three days.

Tokutomi et al. identified that maintaining a temperature range of 35-35.5°C effectively managed intracranial hypertension without causing cardiac dysfunction. While the precise mechanisms by which hypothermia aids TBI treatment remain unclear, mild TH has been consistently associated with the regulation of proteins such as connexin-43 and glutamate-transporter-1 in the hippocampus following TBI in rat models. Additionally, TH was found to alleviate brain swelling and neurological deficits induced by TBI, potentially through the modulation of connexin-43 expression, which typically increases under normal post-TBI conditions. In line with earlier findings, using a fluid percussion injury model demonstrated that post-traumatic hypothermia significantly reduced cell death in the hippocampus and decreased caspase-3 activation, thereby lowering markers of apoptosis.

Numerous investigations have been conducted to explore the positive effects of therapeutic hypothermia in single-center settings. Polderman provided a summary and review of these recent studies, concluding that mild hypothermia may serve as an effective treatment option for neurological injuries, though further research is warranted. A multicenter randomized controlled trial, led by Clifton et al. known as NAVIS-H (North American

Brain Injury Study; Hypothermia), was launched to assess the benefits of mild hypothermia in treating a substantial cohort of patients with severe traumatic brain injury (TBI). Conducted between 1994 and 1998, the study involved 392 adult patients who were divided into two groups: 193 in the normothermia group and 199 in the hypothermia group. Unlike earlier single-center studies, this larger trial did not demonstrate a significant benefit of hypothermia treatment in reducing mortality rates. However, it was noted that in patients under the age of 45, those treated with hypothermia had a lower incidence of poor outcomes (52%) compared to those in the normothermia group (76%). Additionally, patients who presented with a body temperature below 35°C upon admission experienced more favorable results when treated with hypothermia.

Experiments Using Hypothermia in TBI

Clifton et al. were among the first to demonstrate the benefits of moderate hypothermia in treating traumatic brain injury (TBI) using a rat model. Their research showed that maintaining a body temperature of 30°C significantly lowered mortality rates when compared to a control group with normal body temperature. Subsequent studies by Lyeth et al. and Dietrich et al. supported these findings, indicating positive outcomes from moderate hypothermia in animal models of TBI. Additionally, research by Dixon et al. indicated that hypothermia after trauma could decrease the size of brain contusions following a controlled cortical impact. One challenge in applying these findings clinically is identifying the optimal timing for therapeutic interventions. While various drug treatments have proven effective if administered before or immediately following an injury, delayed treatments have not shown similar levels of clinical effectiveness. In exploring the timing for hypothermic treatment, Markgraf et al. found that initiating moderate hypothermia (3 hours at 30°C) within 60 to 90 minutes post-injury led to improved neurological outcomes. The practical application of this narrow time window in clinical settings remains uncertain, particularly whether the timings observed in animal studies will translate effectively to human treatments. Furthermore, studies have demonstrated that post-traumatic hypothermia can mitigate the progression of axonal damage in TBI models. Given the critical role of diffuse axonal injury (DAI) in the functional impairments associated with TBI, these results underscore the potential importance of therapeutic hypothermia in managing TBI.

The Pathophysiology of Trapeutic Hypothermia in Traumatic Brain Injury

The beneficial impacts of hypothermia were once attributed primarily to its metabolic and energy conservation effects. Recent research over the past ten years, however, has shown that even mild hypothermic conditions can counteract various processes that contribute to secondary brain injury. This type of injury begins at the time of the initial trauma and continues to develop in the subsequent minutes, hours, and days, significantly influencing both the prognosis and the effectiveness of treatments for patients. The exact pathophysiological mechanisms that drive this secondary damage remain elusive.

In terms of the broader impacts on brain injury, several biomolecular and physiological alterations could play a role. These include neuroinflammatory responses marked by cytokine release, the production of excitotoxic agents, the formation of cerebral edema, elevated intracranial pressure (ICP), and reduced cerebral blood flow, which may lead to ischemia and cell death through apoptosis. Hypothermia moderates slight changes in brain temperature that occur during or after an ischemic or traumatic event, potentially altering hemodynamic responses. Furthermore, it affects excitatory calcium-dependent signaling between cells, inflammation, edema, apoptosis, and various molecular indicators in the brain following injury. Initial research indicated that mild post-traumatic hypothermia reduces extracellular levels of glutamate and other excitatory neurotransmitters. This mild cooling of the body also aids in safeguarding the blood-brain barrier from increased permeability, which typically follows ischemic and traumatic injuries to tight cerebral capillaries. Such increased permeability can cause brain edema, potentially due to cell membrane damage from hypoxia, which leads to swelling of brain cells, as well as the presence of cytotoxic and excitatory agents.

One significant benefit of hypothermia is its role in maintaining the integrity of the blood-brain barrier, countering the adverse effects of ischemia-reperfusion, traumatic impacts, or treatments like mannitol administration. Furthermore, hypothermia helps mitigate the release of nitric oxide (NO), which can enhance vascular permeability in brain endothelial cells, reduce recruitment of neuronal NO synthase, and diminish aquaporin-4 expression.

Recent findings suggest that hypothermia affects signaling pathways related to hippocampal-dependent learning and memory functions, potentially revealing a molecular mechanism through which hypothermia treatment improves functional outcomes following traumatic brain injury.

Overall, hypothermia provides a protective shield against various harmful mechanisms in the brain after events such as ischemia-reperfusion or trauma. Initially, these protective effects include reductions in cerebral metabolism, mitochondrial damage, ion pump malfunctions, and excitotoxicity. In later stages, it can also lessen reperfusion injuries, reactive oxygen species (ROS) production, inflammation, apoptosis, issues with blood-brain barrier integrity, and edema.

Additionally, hypothermia plays a role in neuronal cell regeneration and the repair of neuronal circuits. Therefore, the capacity of temperature management post-brain injury to influence immediate and subsequent biochemical and genetic responses has broadened our comprehension of the complex effects temperature can have on pathophysiology and recovery processes [50].

Conclusion and Suggestions

Studies on hypothermia commenced in the 1950s, and it has since been understood that its impacts extend beyond merely decelerating metabolism and lowering brain oxygen usage. Approximately four decades ago, the European Resuscitation Council and the American Heart Association first advocated mild hypothermia as a therapeutic measure following cardiac arrest [51]. They advised that patients who regain spontaneous circulation post-resuscitation specifically those with an initial rhythm of ventricular fibrillation and who remain unconscious—should have their body temperature reduced to between 32-34°C for 12-24 hours. This cooling process might also be beneficial for other cardiac rhythms or arrests occurring within hospital settings.

It is critical to treat hypothermia akin to a pharmacological agent, with vigilant monitoring of body temperature throughout its application. Advances in rapid cooling techniques have led to a preference for esophageal temperature monitoring over bladder monitoring due to the former's quicker responsiveness in reflecting changes in core body temperature. Despite the established knowledge regarding hypothermia's role, there is a need for additional research to ascertain the most effective depth and length of cooling, the ideal rewarming rate for patients, and the various methods for initiating hypothermia. Experimental studies involving primates are also suggested to explore hypothermia's function during cardiopulmonary resuscitation and prior to the return of spontaneous circulation. The utility of mild hypothermia is well recognized in cases of cardiac arrest, yet there is potential for its application in conditions such as stroke, traumatic brain injury, myocardial infarction, hemorrhagic shock, renal failure, pulmonary failure, or sepsis. These areas present promising opportunities for further investigation and should be prioritized in future research endeavors. As patient survival and recovery rates from cardiac arrest improve, public satisfaction with emergency medical services and hospitals is likely to rise, enhancing the community's perception of medical facilities.

References

[1] Bouch D, Thompson J, Damian M. *Post-cardiac arrest management: more than global cooling?*: Oxford University Press; 2008. p. 591-4.

[2] Halabchi F, Seif-Barghi T, Mazaheri R. Sudden cardiac death in young athletes; a literature review and special considerations in Asia. *Asian journal of sports medicine*. 2011;2(1):1.

[3] Behringer W, Bernard S, Holzer M, Polderman K, Tiaineu M, Roine RO. Prevention of postresuscitation neurologic dysfunction and injury by the use of therapeutic mild hypothermia. *Cardiac arrest–the science and practice of resusciation medicine* Cambridge University Press, Cambridge. 2007:848-84.

[4] Fairbanks RJ, Shah MN, Lerner EB, Ilangovan K, Pennington EC, Schneider SM. Epidemiology and outcomes of out-of-hospital cardiac arrest in Rochester, New York. *Resuscitation*. 2007;72(3):415-24.

[5] Bernard SA, Gray TW, Buist MD, Jones BM, Silvester W, Gutteridge G, et al. Treatment of comatose survivors of out-of-hospital cardiac arrest with induced hypothermia. *New England journal of medicine*. 2002;346(8):557-63.

[6] Sterz F, Holzer M, Roine R, Zeiner A, Losert H, Eisenburger P, et al. Hypothermia after cardiac arrest: a treatment that works. *Current opinion in critical care*. 2003;9(3):205-10.

[7] Soleimanpour H, Gholipouri C, Salarilak S, Raoufi P, Vahidi RG, Rouhi AJ, et al. Emergency department patient satisfaction survey in Imam Reza hospital, Tabriz, Iran. *International journal of emergency medicine*. 2011;4:1-7.

[8] Foëx BA, Butler J. Therapeutic hypothermia after out of hospital cardiac arrest. *Emergency Medicine Journal*. 2004;21(5):590-1.

[9] Mahmoodpoor A, Shokouhi G, Hamishehkar H, Soleimanpour H, Sanaie S, Porhomayon J, et al. A pilot trial of l-carnitine in patients with traumatic brain injury: Effects on biomarkers of injury. *Journal of critical care*. 2018;45:128-32.

[10] Hörburger D, Sterz F, Herkner H, Holzer M. Defining the optimal target temperature following cardiac arrest. *Critical care medicine*. 2012;40(11):3118-9.

[11] Soleimanpour H, Gholipouri C, Panahi JR, Afhami MR, Ghafouri RR, Golzari SE, et al. Role of anesthesiology curriculum in improving bag-mask ventilation and intubation success rates of emergency medicine residents: a prospective descriptive study. *BMC emergency medicine*. 2011;11:1-6.

[12] Soleimanpour H, Ziapour B, Negargar S, Taghizadieh A, Shadvar K. Ventricular tachycardia due to flumazenil administration. *Pakistan journal of biological sciences: PJBS*. 2010;13(23):1161-3.

[13] Soleimanpour H, Rahmani F, Safari S, Golzari SE. Hypothermia after cardiac arrest as a novel approach to increase survival in cardiopulmonary cerebral resuscitation: a review. *Iranian Red Crescent Medical Journal.* 2014;16(7):e17497.
[14] Werner LM, Kevorkian CRT, Getnet MD, Rios KE, Hull LDM, Robben CPM, et al. Hypothermia: Pathophysiology and the propensity for infection. The American *Journal of Emergency Medicine.* 2024.
[15] Soleimanpour H, Safari S, Nia KS, Sanaie S, Alavian SM. Opioid drugs in patients with liver disease: a systematic review. *Hepatitis monthly.* 2016;16(4):e32636.
[16] Miner J, Tintinalli J, Stapczynski J, Cline D, Ma O, Cydulka R, et al. Procedural sedation and analgesia. *Tintinalli's Emergency Medicine.* 2011:283-91.
[17] Soleimanpour H, Taheraghdam A, Ghafouri RR, Taghizadieh A, Marjany K, Soleimanpour M. Improvement of refractory migraine headache by propofol: case series. *International Journal of Emergency Medicine.* 2012;5:1-4.
[18] Soleimanpour H, Ghafouri RR, Taheraghdam A, Aghamohammadi D, Negargar S, Golzari SE, et al. Effectiveness of intravenous dexamethasone versus propofol for pain relief in the migraine headache: a prospective double blind randomized clinical trial. *BMC neurology.* 2012;12:1-7.
[19] Soleymanpour H, Marjani K, Iranpour A, Rajaei Gr, Soleymanpour M. *The Comparison of Propofol and Nesdonal On Succinylcholine-Induced Fasciculations, Myalgia and Postoperative Sore Throat.* 2009.
[20] Ghojazadeh M, Sanaie S, Paknezhad SP, Faghih S-S, Soleimanpour H. Using ketamine and propofol for procedural sedation of adults in the emergency department: a systematic review and meta-analysis. *Advanced Pharmaceutical Bulletin.* 2019;9(1):5.
[21] Dronen SC. Pharmacologic adjuncts to intubation. *Clinical Procedures in Emergency Medicine* Philadelphia, PA: WB Saunders. 1998:45-57.
[22] Soleimanpour H, Khoshnudi F, Movaghar M, Ziapour B. Improvement of decerebrate status in a hanged child following emergent tracheostomy. *Pakistan journal of biological sciences: PJBS.* 2010;13(23):1164-5.
[23] Soleimanpour H, Sarahrudi K, Hadju S, Golzari S. How to overcome difficult-bag-mask-ventilation: Recents approaches. *Emerg Med.* 2012;2(04).
[24] Soleimanpour H, Gholipouri C, Golzari SE, Rahmani F, Sabahi M, Mottram AR. Capnography in the emergency department. *Emergency Med.* 2012;2(09):10.4172.
[25] Al-Senani FM, Graffagnino C, Grotta JC, Saiki R, Wood D, Chung W, et al. A prospective, multicenter pilot study to evaluate the feasibility and safety of using the CoolGard™ System and Icy™ catheter following cardiac arrest. *Resuscitation.* 2004;62(2):143-50.
[26] Soleimanpour H, Panahi J, Mahmoodpoor A, Ghafouri RR. Digital intubation training in residency program, as an alternative method in airway management. *Pak J Med Sci.* 2011;27(2):401-4.
[27] Lüsebrink E, Binzenhöfer L, Kellnar A, Scherer C, Schier J, Kleeberger J, et al. Targeted temperature management in postresuscitation care after incorporating results of the TTM2 trial. *Journal of the American Heart Association.* 2022;11(21):e026539.

[28] Wolfrum S, Roedl K, Hanebutte A, Pfeifer R, Kurowski V, Riessen R, et al. Temperature control after in-hospital cardiac arrest: a randomized clinical trial. *Circulation.* 2022;146(18):1357-66.

[29] Doerning R, Danielson KR, Hall J, Counts CR, Sayre MR, Wahlster S, et al. Targeted Temperature Management At 33 Versus 36 Degrees After Out-Of-Hospital Cardiac Arrest: A Follow-Up Study. *Resuscitation Plus.* 2025:100921.

[30] Kumar D, Tran K, Premji Z. Temperature Management in Patients After Cardiac Arrest: *CADTH Health Technology Review.* 2023.

[31] NOZARI A. Mild therapeutic hypothermia to improve the neurologic outcome after cardiac arrest. *50 Studies Every Intensivist Should Know.* 2018:1.

[32] Arrich J, Holzer M, Herkner H, Müllner M. Hypothermia for neuroprotection in adults after cardiopulmonary resuscitation. *Anesthesia & Analgesia.* 2010;110(4):1239.

[33] Group W, Nolan J, Morley P, Vanden Hoek T, Hickey R, Force ALST, et al. Therapeutic hypothermia after cardiac arrest: an advisory statement by the advanced life support task force of the International Liaison Committee on Resuscitation. *Circulation.* 2003;108(1):118-21.

[34] Holzer M, Müllner M, Sterz F, Robak O, Kliegel A, Losert H, et al. Efficacy and safety of endovascular cooling after cardiac arrest: cohort study and Bayesian approach. *Stroke.* 2006;37(7):1792-7.

[35] Mooney MR, Unger BT, Boland LL, Burke MN, Kebed KY, Graham KJ, et al. Therapeutic hypothermia after out-of-hospital cardiac arrest: evaluation of a regional system to increase access to cooling. *Circulation.* 2011;124(2):206-14.

[36] Walters JH, Morley PT, Nolan JP. The role of hypothermia in post-cardiac arrest patients with return of spontaneous circulation: a systematic review. *Resuscitation.* 2011;82(5):508-16.

[37] Dixon S, Whitbourn R, Dae M. Induction of mild systemic hypothermia with endovascular cooling during primary percutaneous coronary intervention for acute myocardial infarction. *ACC Current Journal Review.* 2003;12(2):76.

[38] Kang IS, Fumiaki I, Pyun WB. Therapeutic hypothermia for cardioprotection in acute myocardial infarction. *Yonsei Medical Journal.* 2016;57(2):291.

[39] Jung KT, Bapat A, Kim YK, Hucker WJ, Lee K. Therapeutic hypothermia for acute myocardial infarction: a narrative review of evidence from animal and clinical studies. *Korean Journal of Anesthesiology.* 2022;75(3):216-30.

[40] Kohlhauer M, Berdeaux A, Ghaleh B, Tissier R. Therapeutic hypothermia to protect the heart against acute myocardial infarction. *Archives of cardiovascular diseases.* 2016;109(12):716-22.

[41] Yamada KP, Kariya T, Aikawa T, Ishikawa K. Effects of therapeutic hypothermia on normal and ischemic heart. *Frontiers in Cardiovascular Medicine.* 2021;8:642843.

[42] Nanchal R, Kumar G. *Hypothermia in Acute Liver Failure.* Edited by Farid Sadaka. 2013:99.

[43] Felberg R, Krieger D, Chuang Ra, Persse D, Burgin W, Hickenbottom S, et al. Hypothermia after cardiac arrest: feasibility and safety of an external cooling protocol. *Circulation.* 2001;104(15):1799-804.

[44] Stravitz RT, Lee WM, Kramer AH, Kramer DJ, Hynan L, Blei AT. Therapeutic hypothermia for acute liver failure: toward a randomized, controlled trial in patients with advanced hepatic encephalopathy. *Neurocritical care.* 2008;9:90-6.

[45] Vaquero J. Therapeutic hypothermia in the management of acute liver failure. *Neurochemistry international.* 2012;60(7):723-35.

[46] Gharizadeh N, Ghojazadeh M, Naseri A, Dolati S, Tarighat F, Soleimanpour H. Hypertonic saline for traumatic brain injury: a systematic review and meta-analysis. *European Journal of Medical Research.* 2022;27(1):254.

[47] You JS, Kim JY, Yenari MA. Therapeutic hypothermia for stroke: Unique challenges at the bedside. *Frontiers in Neurology.* 2022;13:951586.

[48] Chen H, Wu F, Yang P, Shao J, Chen Q, Zheng R. A meta-analysis of the effects of therapeutic hypothermia in adult patients with traumatic brain injury. *Critical Care.* 2019;23:1-12.

[49] Andresen M, Gazmuri JT, Marín A, Regueira T, Rovegno M. Therapeutic hypothermia for acute brain injuries. *Scandinavian journal of trauma, resuscitation and emergency medicine.* 2015;23:1-7.

[50] Kim DK, Hyun DK. Therapeutic Hypothermia in Traumatic Brain injury; Review of History, Pathophysiology and Current Studies. *Korean Journal of Critical Care Medicine.* 2015;30(3):143-50.

[51] Uray T, Haugk M, Sterz F, Arrich J, Richling N, Janata A, et al. Surface cooling for rapid induction of mild hypothermia after cardiac arrest: design determines efficacy. *Academic Emergency Medicine.* 2010;17(4):360-7.

About the Authors

Hassan Soleimanpour
  Emergency and Trauma Care Research Center
  Imam Reza General Hospital
  Tabriz University of Medical Sciences
  Tabriz, Iran

Tannaz Novinbahador
  Immunology Research Center
  Tabriz University of Medical Sciences
  Tabriz, Iran

Farzad Rahmani
  Emergency and Trauma Care Research Center
  Imam Reza General Hospital
  Tabriz University of Medical Sciences
  Tabriz, Iran

Index

A

acute coronary syndrome, 37
acute liver failure (ALF), xx, 73, 74, 75, 76, 77, 78, 79, 80, 81, 101, 102
acute myocardial infarction (AMI), xx, 61, 62, 63, 64, 65, 70, 101
adverse effects, 5, 29, 49, 57, 59, 91, 92, 95
alcohol baths, 42
anesthesia depth, 38
anticoagulant effect, 18
apoptosis, 6, 8, 63, 83, 84, 85, 93, 95, 96
arrhythmias, 15, 16, 17, 26, 59, 92
atracurium, 31, 32

B

bispectral index (BIS), xxi, 38
blood circulation, 2, 37
blood gas levels, 17, 18
blood pressure, xix, 14, 25, 30, 31, 37, 42, 53
blood-brain barrier, xix, 7, 8, 55, 57, 95, 96
body cavity lavage, 46
brain glucose metabolism, 77
brain injuries, xiii, xvii, 10, 11, 24, 59, 74, 85, 102
brain metabolism, 6, 9, 83
brain temperature, 1, 9, 83, 88, 95

C

calpain-related proteolysis, 6
capnography, 35, 36, 37, 100
cardiac arrest, xiii, xiv, xvii, xix, xx, 1, 3, 5, 6, 7, 9, 10, 16, 24, 25, 26, 29, 35, 36, 37, 38, 41, 42, 43, 47, 48, 49, 50, 53, 55, 56, 57, 58, 59, 61, 62, 73, 97, 99, 100, 101, 102
cardiogenic shock, 25, 49, 69
cardioprotective mechanisms, 66
cardiopulmonary bypass, xx, 44
cardiopulmonary resuscitation, xiii, xvii, xix, xx, 1, 10, 36, 37, 56, 60, 97, 101
cardiovascular effects, 1, 14
carotid arteries, 47
cell death, 6, 7, 84, 85, 93, 95
cell survival, 85
cerebral blood flow (CBF), xxi, 10, 14, 75, 76, 77, 79, 83, 92, 95
cerebral resuscitation, xiii, xx, 37, 56, 100
chilled intravenous fluid, 13, 37, 60
cis-atracurium, 32
coagulation, 1, 10, 18, 23
coagulative activity, 10
comas, xiii
cooling cap, 42
core body temperature, xix, 2, 9, 15, 18, 19, 21, 22, 25, 38, 42, 43, 45, 46, 48, 53, 54, 56, 60, 61, 97
coronary blood flow, 15
criteria for exclusion, 25

D

defibrillation, xvii, 43
drug metabolism, 13, 23, 59

E

edema, 8, 38, 42, 43, 54, 55, 57, 75, 76, 77, 78, 79, 80, 91, 92, 95, 96

electrocardiogram, 14, 26, 37
electroencephalogram (EEG), 39
electrolyte disturbances, 16, 17
electrolyte imbalances, 13, 15, 17, 59, 74
electromyography, 39
eligibility criteria, 25
EMcools pad, 42, 58
emergency cooling system, 42
endotracheal tube, 35, 36, 37
energy preservation, 66
extracellular acidosis, 9
extracorporeal membrane oxygenation, xx

F

fentanyl, 23, 27, 28, 29
Food and Drug Administration (FDA), 39
free radicals, 7, 8, 55, 57

H

heart attacks, xiii
hemodynamic changes, 14
hemodynamics, x, 29, 30, 76, 77, 80, 81
hepatic encephalopathy, xiii, 77, 102
hydrogen peroxide, 8
hydroxyl radicals, 8
hyperglycemia, 17, 23, 59, 93
hypoxic brain injury, xvii

I

ice water, 42
ice-cold perfluorocarbon ventilation, 45
immune function, 7, 18, 19, 21
immune response, 7, 8, 86
immune system, 7, 86
immunosuppression, 21
infection, 1, 18, 19, 20, 22, 88, 100
inflammatory response, 7, 18, 21, 63, 76, 86
intensive care unit, xvii, 5, 16, 19, 23, 41
interleukin-1, 7
intracellular acidosis, 9
intravascular cooling, 43, 49, 58, 60
intravenous cold fluid, xix, 42, 60

ion pumps, 6, 9
ischemia, 6, 7, 8, 9, 10, 15, 26, 55, 57, 63, 64, 65, 66, 67, 68, 74, 84, 85, 86, 87, 95, 96

M

mechanical ventilation, 13, 17, 18, 21, 35
meperidine, 27, 29, 45
metabolic effects, 17
metabolism, 6, 13, 17, 23, 30, 36, 57, 63, 66, 75, 77, 84, 92, 96, 97
microvascular obstruction, 65, 68
midazolam, 29, 35
mild hypothermia, xiii, 1, 10, 13, 14, 20, 22, 27, 41, 42, 49, 53, 56, 60, 61, 63, 64, 65, 66, 68, 75, 78, 79, 80, 81, 83, 84, 85, 87, 91, 93, 97, 99, 102
mitochondria, 30, 66, 67, 84
mitochondrial dysfunction, 6
morphine, 27, 28, 29
mortality, xiii, 1, 9, 16, 17, 19, 21, 22, 49, 51, 55, 56, 59, 61, 62, 65, 75, 81, 87, 91, 92, 94
muscle relaxants, 23, 27, 31, 32, 33, 35, 41, 45, 48, 54

N

neurological impairment, xvii, 23, 43, 50
neurological outcomes, xiii, 1, 5, 9, 10, 13, 16, 37, 42, 45, 48, 49, 53, 55, 56, 57, 58, 61, 62, 74, 91, 92, 94
neuronal excitation, 6
neuronal injury, 55
neurotensin, 45, 46
non-convulsive seizures, 11

O

opioids, 27, 28, 29
osmotic balance, 76, 78
oxygen deprivation, xvii

P

pancuronium, 31
patient assessment, 35
peroxynitrite, 8
pethidine, 27, 87
pharmacokinetics, 23, 30
pharmacological interventions, xvii
pharmacological techniques, 44
post-reperfusion, 6, 67, 68
post-resuscitation, xiii, xvii, 6, 25, 97
propofol, 23, 30, 37, 100
prostaglandin E2 (PGE2), xix, 10

R

reactive oxygen species, xx, 63, 67, 85, 96
remifentanil, 28, 29
resuscitation, xiii, xvii, xix, 3, 6, 10, 24, 25, 35, 36, 43, 48, 50, 53, 55, 56, 97, 99, 100, 101, 102
rewarming, 2, 13, 14, 15, 44, 53, 54, 56, 58, 64, 70, 97

S

sedatives, 23, 27, 28, 29, 37, 41, 44, 48, 53
seizure activities, 11, 80
sepsis, 2, 20, 21, 22, 26, 49, 56, 59, 97
shivering, 1, 13, 22, 23, 27, 35, 41, 44, 48, 53, 59, 87
signaling pathways, 68, 95
STEMI-related cardiogenic shock, 69
stroke(s), xiii, 8, 9, 18, 24, 26, 56, 61, 80, 83, 84, 85, 86, 87, 88, 89, 91, 97, 101, 102
sudden cardiac death, xvii, 99
sufentanil, 29
superoxide, 8
surface cooling, 1, 13, 41, 62, 71, 88, 102

T

therapeutic hypothermia, xiii, xx, 1, 5, 13, 19, 20, 41, 49, 50, 55, 59, 61, 62, 63, 66, 68, 69, 70, 76, 78, 80, 81, 83, 84, 85, 86, 87, 88, 89, 91, 92, 93, 94, 99, 101, 102
thromboxane A2 (TXA2), xix, 10
tissue plasminogen activator (r-tPA), xix, 10, 18
trans nasal cooling device, 44
traumatic brain injury (TBI), xxi, 5, 8, 9, 15, 18, 73, 91, 92, 93, 94, 95, 96, 97, 99, 102
tumor necrosis factor-alpha, 7, 55

U

unconscious, xiii, 3, 50, 56, 97

V

vascular permeability, 8, 55, 57, 95
vasoconstrictors, 10
vecuronium, 32